One Drop of Rain

Creating a Wave of Colon Cancer Awareness

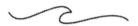

MOLLY MCMASTER MORGOSLEPOV

Courageous

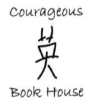

Book House

First Edition

Edited by Karen Bjornland
Cover Design by Troy Burns, Graphic Acuity

ISBN: 978-0-578-45906-6

DEDICATION

I believe that everyone and everything has a place and time in one's life and that they appear for a reason. So many people have helped me on my journey - so many lives have touched mine. I wish I could name them all. People tell me that I'm strong and brave and have done amazing things, but I was just an angry kid surrounded by an incredible bunch of people. This book is dedicated to those people. Thank you for helping me to become the person that I am today.
You are forever in my heart.

In memory of Dr. Orlando J. Martelo

CONTENTS

PART III – MY FIGHT AGAINST CANCER

One Drop of Rain

Creating a Wave of Colon Cancer Awareness

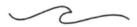

PROLOGUE

"**G**ood morning, Miss Molly. How are you feeling?" Dr. Thompson said. It was February 19, 1999, and I had been in a hospital bed for seven days. I punched the off button on the tiny television hanging from the long robotic arm in front of me and watched him pull the curtain around my bed. He hadn't done that before. The girl in the next bed could hear everything he was going to say anyway, and at that point, nothing could have embarrassed me. I'd already been asked every humiliating question I could imagine, worn the ugly, backless hospital gown for a week, and been poked and prodded in every orifice of my body. I wondered what could possibly warrant a closed-curtain conversation.

"Hi, Dr. Thompson. I'm fine. Did you come to sing "Happy Birthday? I'm 23 today, you know."

"Happy Birthday," he said softly, "But no, not exactly."

"When can I go home?" I asked from my hospital bed in upstate New York but thinking about my trip to

Daytona Beach in less than a week. Rob, my older brother, was in flight school there, and I would be joining my parents for a visit. I couldn't remember the last time we had all taken a family trip.

"Well, I need to talk to you about something." He wasn't smiling, but then again, it wasn't often that I'd seen him smile. I grew up down the street from this man of few words, and it had taken me years to grasp his dry sense of humor. His lips were usually tight, with a slight crook upward on both sides, as if to say, "I'm up to something." But the face he wore this morning was somehow different from the one I was used to seeing.

He walked toward me, and the bed creaked as he sat down on the edge of the mattress.

"Did you run already this morning?" I asked, trying to sidetrack him. I wasn't quite ready for medical talk at this early hour.

"Not yet," he said. "I'll run later."

I loved how he said it like that, so nonchalant. He belonged to a somewhat legendary running group that met *every single day* -- rain, snow, sleet or shine -- in the parking lot of the local YMCA. Dr. Thompson himself had run more marathons than I cared to count, which was pure insanity to me, but to him it was just another day. The man definitely loved his routine.

"Molly, you understand what has happened, right?" He looked so serious and yet somehow more unsure of himself with every word.

"I think so," I replied.

"OK. Let me go over it with you, just to be sure." I nodded and waited for him to continue, but he took his time while I smiled, still thinking of the group of older men trotting through town on the same roads day after day.

"We removed a tumor from your large intestine." He took a breath and blew it out. "The tumor was extremely large, the size of my two fists." He held his fists together in front of me, and I stopped wondering how many pairs of sneakers Dr. Thompson owned and started wondering what that pink, wet, messy blob really looked like. "It was a total obstruction, which is why you were in so much pain."

"Right." I nodded, trying to appear calm and composed.

"We took out about twenty-five inches of large intestine, along with the tumor," he continued, while I pictured it all coiled up like a snake in a jar, smelling strongly of antiseptic.

"And we did some testing here at our lab and also sent out some slides to a national research center, just to be sure."

I nodded, pretending to follow. "Yup."

He looked into my eyes. "Molly, we thought your tumor was going to be benign, but it wasn't."

"OK," I said calmly, but the tight-lipped smile showed him that I hadn't comprehended quite yet.

He took another long, slow breath. "It was colon cancer."

Suddenly, his chilly hand holding mine felt like boiling water. I tried to yank it away but couldn't escape his grasp.

"I've referred you to Dr. Orlando Martelo..."

Cancer.

My face was hot, and tears began to burn my cheeks. Didn't everyone who got cancer die? And lose their hair? Everyone would know I was sick. How could this have happened to me? I wanted to disappear. I wanted to die. I was going to die.

3

"You'll want to get a second opinion…"

I pictured myself as if in a movie scene, stepping gently into thin air from a huge dusty rock, falling down, down, down, and then landing with a thud on another rock below. I watched myself gasping for air that I couldn't find, bleeding and crying out in pain.

My movie quickly cut to a new scene where I stood alone in a bathroom. The reflection staring back at me had a mostly shiny scalp, with bits of fuzz standing up in odd directions. My right hand held a gun, but with the same quickness as the first scene had changed, the gun faded from my hand the moment I realized that I didn't own a gun or have access to one. Now my empty hand reached toward a foggy glass door and gently opened it to reveal a half-empty medicine cabinet. I pulled out a prescription bottle and watched myself pushing down and twisting the cap.

Again, the scene quickly changed. This time, crisp sterile walls surrounded me, and sharp, white overhead lights burned my eyes. My clothes and cheeks were vomit-stained and what looked like black ink that someone had tried to wipe away had spread around the outside of my mouth and across my cheek. I choked as blue latex fingertips thrust a thick tube down my throat.

My movie clicked like the old slideshow Dad used to put on in the living room. In the next scene, I was sitting fully-clothed in a bathtub. The sleeve of my left arm had been rolled up to expose my wrist, and in my right hand was Mom's black-handled KitchenAid paring knife. My hands were shaking and tears wouldn't stop coming as I pressed the blade to my wrist but only left a scratch. More tears. I tried again but couldn't slide the knife and press all at once. On my third attempt, my slideshow clicked once again.

This time it was dark. I was in our garage. The steering wheel of Mom's bronze Honda Accord brushed my knees and the engine was humming. I looked over my shoulder at the door into the house and saw Dr. Thompson standing in the doorway in his bright, white doctor coat. He was still talking.

"...and we've talked to Dana-Farber. Dr. Martelo has referred..."

In this final scene of my movie, I leaned my head slowly back against the headrest, closed my eyes and breathed the toxic air.

PART I

BEFORE CANCER

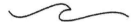

"The greatest accomplishment in life is not in never falling, but in rising again after the fall."

Vincent Lombardi

1

LESSON ONE

♦

The first time I heard about colon cancer was during Mr. Mulvany's health class at Glens Falls High School. Mr. Mulvany limped through the rows of desks while clicking through a slide show on the big, white, pull-down screen at the front of the room. My brother had been in his class four or five years earlier and once told me that he limped because one leg was shorter than the other. I looked down at Mr. Mulvany's feet as he passed and wondered how Rob had that kind of information. Rob knew how to get anything – extra lunch money from a friend, keys to my parents' car, an extra day or two to get a report finished – and the teachers loved him. He had been voted the class mooch when he graduated in 1989, and he did the title proud.

"Pooping once a day helps prevent colon cancer," Mr. Mulvany announced to a classroom of students who were much amused and filled with teenage hormones. My eyes snapped back to the screen. My classmates and I cringed at the grossly distorted red blob, an image that supposedly represented colon cancer. Then, with a click of the projector and the appearance of a new blob, Mr. Mulvany moved on to liver disease.

That was the beginning of what would become my extensive education about colon cancer, but as I left health class that day, my worries about not "pooping once a day" quickly faded.

"Hey, Moe!" Kristina shouted across the hallway after the final bell. It was the same nickname she had called me since around the second or third grade. "You comin' over?"

I'd lived around the corner from Kristina since I was five years old, which was when my father accepted a new job and my family moved from New Jersey to Glens Falls, New York, a small town near the Adirondack Mountains. She was the first person I had met, and I couldn't remember a single day when we hadn't at least spoken on the phone. We had done just about everything together, from figure skating lessons at age seven, to skipping school to take a day-long drive. Multiple times we were caught huddled in a dark closet trying to pierce my ears with an ice cube and needle. I had always been jealous of her pierced ears, and she, being a true friend, just wanted to help. It was hard to imagine leaving her when I went away to college in the fall.

"I've got to start my college applications and write an essay," I said unhappily.

"Oooh. Anything interesting?"

"I have to write about what I want to do with my life."

"They want to know about your bank robber aspirations?"

"Very funny."

That afternoon, when I sat down to write my college essay, I found myself staring at the paper as fear enveloped me.

I wanted to major in English and move to Colorado where the snow was light, the mountains were immense, and rumor was that there were cowboys in every class. It was a place where I could meet new people, see new things, take risks, fall in love and have my heart broken. It was a place where I wouldn't worry about what anyone else thought of me, and I could grow happily into my own skin.

But back in reality, sitting at my desk and fighting writer's block, I was terrified of failing and of disappointing anyone. I was terrified of taking that chance. My dream was to go to college and learn to write books and short stories that would make people love, laugh and cry. But wouldn't life be easier if I stayed close to home? Mom and Dad would be nearby and would help whenever I needed them.

In the spring, I was relieved to receive acceptance letters to Lyndon State and Green Mountain College, the only two schools to which I'd applied.

Mom broke the silence over dinner one night.

"So, have you chosen?"

I was still stewing over an episode earlier that day at the bank.

"Are you Trudie's daughter?" the teller had cooed. My mother sold real estate and her name seemed to be all over town. The bank teller's question was one I got at least once a week and was a constant reminder of how invisible I was.

"I think I want to go to Green Mountain," I answered.

"Oh, Molly. Are you sure?" Her voice sounded so disappointed. "It's so small, and it's so close."

Green Mountain was in Vermont, a mere 32 miles from Glens Falls, and its student body was about 500, roughly half the size of my high school. The truth was that a forty-five-minute drive home was a lot more appealing than the four-hour drive to Lyndon in northern Vermont, and I was already planning to come home on weekends.

"I'm sure," I replied.

As my friends and I spent the summer saying our goodbyes, I imagined how our lives would take many of the same twists and turns even though we were in different geographic places. I had no idea how different my map would be.

I met Christian in my first semester of college, in the lounge of my dorm. He was so cool. He walked like he was wearing an Armani suit and had a million bucks in his pocket, even though he was wearing ripped jeans and a white, fitted cotton undershirt. It was probably a good day for him if he was carrying a five-dollar bill. When I first laid eyes on him, my stomach turned over.

"Hi," he said with a smirk. Goosebumps ran up my neck. He was lean and handsome, a little bit taller than me, with loose dark hair that fell around his eyes.

"Hi," I said, slightly embarrassed that he caught me staring. With that one flirty semi-smile, he became my first college crush.

In the following weeks, I found a sudden interest in rugby and coerced my friends into attending his games and parties in hopes of getting the chance to see him. I made friends with his friends and began working my way into his circle.

Like me, Christian was an English major, but much more the artsy kind. He was a junior, played the guitar and piano, wrote poetry and didn't seem to care what anyone thought about him, a trait I admired beyond comprehension. To him, I was probably just an annoying freshman, but he humored me and let me follow him around when he was free. When he talked, I listened intently, and I pretended not to notice that he rarely asked about me.

"What do you want to do when you finish school?" I asked him innocently one afternoon while sitting cross-legged on a couch and listening as he played the Journey song "Faithfully" on the piano. It was a question I always asked friends, in hopes that someone might be as confused about life as I was. I should have known better.

"I'm going to be an actor on Broadway."

"No, really." I laughed.

"Really," he said, taking his fingers from the keys abruptly, obviously annoyed at my reaction.

"Wow. I don't think I've ever known anyone who wanted to be an actor."

"I'll go to grad school when I finish here, and then I'll move to New York City and go to as many auditions as I can find."

I smiled. "I can picture that," I said. "What about TV?"

He shook his head. "Broadway," he repeated. "I'll never do any of that soap opera crap."

"You're going to be a great actor," I told him, partly just to feed his ego. "Can I have your autograph so that someday when you're famous ..."

"Very funny," he interrupted, putting his fingers back to the keys.

The fall semester came to a close, and as I packed the last of my things into my red Jeep Wrangler in the cold rain, I watched Christian walk across the snowy campus hand-in-hand with his new, very blond and very beautiful girlfriend. He was dating his co-star in the school's fall production, and my time with him had become hers. A sickening disappointment enveloped me as they disappeared through the doors of the dining hall.

I silently scolded myself for not being confident enough to tell him how I felt earlier in the semester, all the while losing sight of my own bigger picture. I had wanted Colorado. I had settled for Vermont. I slipped behind the wheel of my Jeep, slid the key into the ignition, and simultaneously slipped out from under Christian's spell.

Back at school at the end of January, I felt a strange new beginning. My new schedule was busy and active, and I got back to my old routine of working out five days a week. In the spring, when the snow began to melt, I started in-line skating. I always loved to skate and found that it allowed me to be alone with my thoughts every day. I liked what I was finding. I liked *who* I was finding. Each day, I seemed to gain a bit more confidence. My dream was on the horizon again. If I was ever going to meet the *real* Molly, I had to get out of the "little pond," and I finally felt ready. Somehow, life in Colorado didn't seem so scary anymore. I was ready to take on the West. I secretly applied to Colorado State University and was accepted as a transfer student for the fall semester.

"I can't believe you're moving to Colorado," Bruce exclaimed. "I'm jealous!" My friend and I were out for a drive back home in Glens Falls one afternoon, shortly after I'd received my acceptance letter.

"I know! It's so far from home, but you can visit me anytime," I told him.

"You know I will! We should celebrate!"

"Ice cream," I exclaimed as the Friendly's sign came into view. It was an unseasonably warm spring day.

"I was thinking more like a Coors Light. You know? Rocky Mountain Water?" He smiled. "Besides, I can't eat ice cream. I'm lactose intolerant."

"What's that?" I asked.

"I'm allergic to dairy," he said. "The stuff does a number on my insides."

"Oh."

"Sucks too, since I love ice cream." He looked at me with an evil grin. "Sometimes I can't help myself and eat the stuff anyway. Man do I pay for it though. I'll spend all night in the bathroom," he said, laughing.

"No ice cream then," I said, rubbing my still pudgy freshman belly. "I'm trying to work it off anyway!"

That night, Bruce's tale of intestinal woe stayed with me, and I convinced myself that I too was lactose intolerant. Something was changing inside of me. I'd been having frequent gas pains and bloating worse than any PMS cramps I'd ever had. I told Mom about my lactose intolerance, and when I went home for a visit the next weekend, there was a half-gallon of lactose-free milk in the refrigerator. Unfortunately, it didn't seem to make a difference, and when I got back to school and found that the cafeteria didn't serve anything lactose-free anyway, I forgot all about it and chalked it up to being a hypochondriac.

When the spring semester finally ended and it was time to say goodbye, I hoped to close the chapter on Christian. He had successfully ignored me through most of the semester, a difficult task on such a small campus, but I wanted to leave on my terms. I knocked on his door.

"Come in," he said.

I pushed the door open into an almost empty room.

"Hi."

"What are you doing here?" There was surprise in his voice, but he seemed to be happy to see me, if only slightly.

"I just wanted to make sure I got the chance to say goodbye."

"That was nice of you," he said genuinely.

"I was also hoping you might write your contact info in here." I handed him a notebook and waited while he scribbled a few lines. "I just…"

"Molly," he interrupted, handing the notebook back to me. "I'm sorry about the way I've been acting toward you." Surprised at his bluntness, I listened quietly.

"I don't know why. I just wasn't sure…" His voice trailed off.

"That's OK." I smiled, not entirely sure what I was supposed to say. "I understand." I really didn't.

"We'll talk more next semester," he continued.

"Well, not exactly. I've been accepted at Colorado State University," I said in my best country cowboy accent. "I'm gonna be a Ram!" A proud smile widened across my lips.

"Oh? That's really great. Long way from home though," he said.

"I know!" I squealed, feeling the butterflies all over again. "I'm really excited! Did you know that Fort Collins boasts 300 days of sunshine a year?"

"I won't be surprised if you're back here within a year," he said matter-of-factly.

I winced at his words, feeling angry and hurt, but stronger than the last time we had spoken. Forcing my smile, I turned and walked out, closing the door gently behind me and holding back tears. The fear of failure was fading. In its place I began to feel rage and a drive to prove that I would not only make it on my own, but that I would be successful and more importantly, happy.

After I left Christian's room, I leaned against a wall and opened my notebook to see what he had written beneath his address.

"Molly, follow the dream. Take it, because no one will give it to you. Take it. Run with it and don't look back. The world is waiting. Don't let it down…."

2

COLORADO

◆

I crammed the last of my most precious belongings into my little red Jeep and drove cross-country with the top down under a hot, July sun. All the way there, I played a James Taylor cassette tape that my friend Sarah had given me the night before I'd left.

"This is a song for you far away, so far away," Taylor crooned. "This is a song for you, far away from me."

As the miles rolled by, and the song played over and over, every single time I heard the words, my heart tightened just a little bit more. What if Colorado was a mistake?

But I arrived in Fort Collins on a flawless day, certain that I'd found paradise, and once again sure of my decision. The mini-metropolis sat slightly southeast of the craggy Poudre Canyon, and at the edge of the Rocky Mountains and Horsetooth Rock, a natural formation that jutted skyward atop the foothills west of town. Longs Peak, one of the 56 mountains in Colorado that stood above 14,000 feet, would be visible every day on my walk to school.

It didn't take long to discover my favorite parts of Colorado -- the mild and misleading weather, and the endless blue sky. After the first dose of snow in early September, I thought it would remain icy cold, but it melted the next day and the temperature was balmy again. As fall came to an end and winter took hold, the days were crisp and breezy, but the sun shone brightly across the huge Colorado sky.

When I arrived in Colorado, I envisioned myself rock climbing, kayaking, mountain biking and skiing, but instead I took up indoor ice hockey. In my hometown, I had been a member of the Glens Falls Figure Skating Club in my younger years and had put many miles on my in-line skates on the roads in Vermont and New York. I always wanted to try hockey. When I found the Fort Collins Flames, a women's ice hockey team, I was hooked instantly.

Unfortunately, I was the slowest skater on the team and didn't know how to stop. Most times, I would just close my eyes and slam into the boards, or another player, and hope for the best. Everyone on the team supposedly got a chance to play, but I was terrible. During games, I played on the fourth line and was shifted every other time around, which meant I was skating, quite literally, every 10 minutes or so, for only about a minute at a time. But I was having the time of my life and making great new friends. I had finally found something that I truly loved, and I wanted to be the best at it that I could possibly be.

In June, I flew back to New York with my in-line skates, hockey stick, gloves and an old tennis ball. My season on the ice had ended, but I was determined to use the off-season to sharpen my skills. I didn't want to just *play* hockey -- I wanted to be *great* at it. Kristina thought I was crazy and just going through a phase, but every day I in-line skated a few miles to build my stamina, and then went home to get my stick and ball to practice stick-handling and shooting.

One morning, I was on my skates after a rain shower. The roads were dry except for a patch here or there under a tree. I zigzagged up the street, passing the ball back and forth between my skates and stick while trying not to roll through a puddle. Suddenly, too focused on the ball, I skated over a wet patch of road and felt my right skate slip out from under me. I couldn't stop myself, and before I knew it, the ball shot across the road and I landed on one knee, then skidded a few feet. I looked up to see two landscapers, very amused by what had happened. I took a breath, stood up and got a glimpse of my knee and a trail of blood that ran all the way into my sock. It stung terribly, but I couldn't let the landscapers see my pain, so I skated over to the grass where the tennis ball had landed, pulled the ball to the pavement with the blade of my hockey stick, and began the whole process again. The two men watched the whole pitiful performance.

After an extra 30 minutes, just to prove how tough I was to two people I didn't even know, I finally skated around the corner to Kristina's house. She helped me clean and bandage my knee and soothe my bruised ego, and I allowed her a few laughs at my expense.

"So, Molly, you really like this hockey stuff, huh?" Dad asked, looking at me in the rearview mirror as he and Mom took me to the airport and my flight back to Colorado.

"Dad, it's *awesome*! I just want to get better and better at it, and I want to practice all the time. Did you know that women's hockey is being added to the '98 Olympics in Nagano next year?"

"Going to play for the Olympics, are you?"

"Maybe someday," I grinned.

"Are you sure it's safe?" Mom asked.

"It's perfectly safe. Mom, when we bump into each other, we all apologize. That seems to be the difference between men's and women's hockey."

"Well, just don't get your teeth knocked out," Dad said. "I don't want to be getting any outrageous dental bills."

"I won't."

"Do you wear a helmet?" Mom asked.

"Of course, I do. We have to," I laughed.

"A face shield?" Dad asked.

"Yup."

"What about a mouth guard?"

"Sure," I lied.

"Well, if it makes you happy, keep playing."

"It does. And I know it sounds crazy, but all I want to do is practice and get better and better. I may even want to be a college coach someday!"

"That's good," he said with slightly more enthusiasm.

"And that's OK with you?" I knew it didn't really matter what his answer was. I was finally living my own life in Colorado, 2,000 miles away. I would still play, even if he told me not to, and he knew that. But Dad had always pushed what he had learned from his own father --- that education was the key to opening every door, and a *good* education with a goal at the end was not only encouraged but expected. I thought back to the night I had told my grandmother about being accepted into the small private college in Vermont. She told me about my cousins who were attending Embry-Riddle Aeronautical University to become commercial airline pilots, and mentioned my brother, who was finishing up at Ithaca College and preparing to do the same. What was I planning to do with myself, she wanted to know.

I caught Dad's eyes in the rearview mirror again. "Molly, I don't care if you collect string," he said, "as long as you do your best and you do it well."

In the fall, when I got back on the ice, the coach didn't even recognize me at our first practice.

"Excuse me," he said, as I skated by during warm-ups. "Did you register?"

I spun around, skated at him full speed, and stopped just before slamming into him, spraying ice up his leg.

"It's me, coach!" I smiled and pulled off my helmet so he could get a good look.

"I'll be damned. You can stop! What happened to you?"

"Practice!" I beamed. "All summer!"

He decided to start me on defense in the first game and most of the rest of the season as well. The next fall, I was thrilled when the team named me as their captain.

I had no idea where kayaking, mountain biking, hiking and skiing had gone, but those were no longer my Colorado dreams. The sweet, salty and sweaty palm of a hockey glove had become one of my favorite smells, and every extra minute was spent on the ice. I was even having dreams of someday playing for the U.S. Women's Olympic Team.

My entire schedule revolved around my love for the game, and I rarely missed the opportunity to get on the ice. On Sunday nights, I played in a men's league, sometimes getting on the ice as late as 11 p.m. After the game, the rink attendant would usually let me stay on the ice and practice alone, sometimes until two a.m. Then I'd head home to do homework or go for a run before driving back to the rink for five a.m. practice with the women's team.

The rest of the week was spent going to class and playing drop-in hockey with the guys. The weekends were reserved for games all over Colorado with the Flames. If we had an away game on Sunday afternoon, I'd rush back to Fort Collins for my Sunday night men's league game. It was an endless cycle and I loved it.

Other than the coaching I got once a week with the women's team, I'd never had any formal hockey training. Sometimes, when I stayed on the ice late at night, some of the guys who worked at the rink, or players from the men's league, would show me something new to work on. That's how I met Rocky.

Late one night after a men's league game, I was doing some skating drills alone when Rocky, still dressed in his equipment from the game, asked if he could join me. I recognized him immediately. I'd met him downtown once before but doubted he remembered me. He had a short, dark-reddish, military-style haircut and baby blue eyes.

Rocky started skating around at the other end of the ice, handling the puck and shooting, but as I skated around the face-off circles and practiced with my own puck, I felt him watching me. Finally, he skated over.

"Can ya roof a backhand?" he asked.

"Roof a backhand?" I asked. "What's that?" I felt stupid not knowing, especially in front of him.

"Can ya take an up-close backhand shot on the goalie and put it over his shoulder and into the top of the net?" His thick Boston accent sounded almost rude.

"Oh," I said. He was obviously amused. "I don't know."

"Lemme see ya try," he said, dropping a puck at my skates and slowly gliding backward. I glanced at the net, only a few feet in front of me, then at Rocky and then back down at the puck.

"OK." I put the heel of my stick on the ice next to the puck, took a deep breath and batted it as hard as I could. The puck rolled sideways pitifully, and into the back of the net.

"That was disgraceful." Rocky laughed.

"Thanks."

By one a.m., I had an 80 percent accurate backhand shot and learned that Rocky was a first lieutenant in the United States Air Force and stationed in Cheyenne, Wyoming, about an hour north of Fort Collins. He was taking graduate classes in environmental engineering at CSU. Unfortunately, Rocky also had a serious girlfriend back in Boston.

Like Christian had been at Green Mountain, Rocky was confident, but he was also silly and always looking for a laugh.

"Hey, Moll," he said in the parking lot after hockey one night.

"Yes, Rock," I answered.

"Did ya hear about the termite that walked into the 'bah'?"

"No, Rock. Please enlighten me."

"Well, this termite walks into a 'bah' and asks the 'bah-tenda,' 'Excuse me, Sir, but is the 'bah *tendah*' here?'" He was already laughing. "Get it? ' Bah – *tendah*?'"

"Very funny, Rock," I threw my bag into the trunk and hopped into the driver's seat of my car. Halfway home, I laughed out loud, finally getting the punchline about the termite looking to chew a tender wooden bar.

Rocky's love for the game and the drive to push himself was something we shared, and he inspired me because he seemed to believe in me. Because his own confidence began rubbing off on me, I started believing in myself.

I was no longer the kid who grew up on Garrison Road constantly hearing "Are you Trudie's daughter?" And it didn't matter that I wasn't a straight A student. My new friends knew *me* for *me* --- Molly, "the chick who plays hockey" and might someday get an invitation to try out for the Women's U.S. Olympic Team. I was excelling at something that I loved, and although it was a small pond, I was becoming a big fish. I was right where I wanted to be.

3

FIRST SYMPTOMS

◊

By the summer of 1998, my third year in Fort Collins, I had started coaching both ice and roller hockey, a warmer version played on wheeled, in-line skates, and I was still very much in love with the game.

In July, much to our shock, Holly, the Flames' starting center, announced that she would be moving at the end of the school year. She and her husband needed someone to watch their four kids, who ranged in age from 4 to 12, while they were in Virginia looking for a place to live. I was already like a fun aunt to the kids, so I was elected for the job.

The morning of their flight, I met Holly to go over the house rules and get acquainted with the kitchen. Holly amazed me. She was 40 years old, had four kids, played hockey, boxed and skied. On our team, she was in better shape than any of us.

"Here's where all the cooking stuff is," she said, opening a cabinet filled with unrecognizable organic ingredients.

"Uh, huh." Certainly she didn't think that a 22-year-old would be cooking meals from scratch for her children.

"There are plenty of snacks in the refrigerator," she continued, opening the fridge door to reveal yogurt, fruit and a jar of granola. "And frozen pizza here." I let out a sigh of relief as she opened the freezer door and I silently counted enough pizza boxes to feed the kids for a week.

"Oh, and there's plenty of beer," she said.

"I'm not a big beer drinker, but thanks for thinking of me."

"Oh, you'll need it," she said with a grin.

Later that afternoon, after Holly and her husband left for the airport, the fun began.

"What do you guys want to do first?"

"Can Xander spend the night?" Maddie asked.

"Let's go for a bike ride," Eliza said.

"Can we watch a movie?" asked Jesse.

"Roller hockey!" Nat exclaimed.

"Great," I said. "How about if we ride our bikes to the movie store and rent something for tonight. I know one you guys will love. Yes, Maddie, Xander can spend the night if it's OK with his mother, and Nat, let's play hockey tomorrow morning when it's cooler. Sound good?" I had this parenting thing down.

Ten minutes later we were all biking single file through the neighborhood.

At the movie store, we rented one of my old favorites, *The Goonies*, and I bought a large bag of gummy bears and some balloons. I figured a game of water balloon toss would keep them occupied for a bit. "This is going to be a breeze," I said under my breath.

But back at the house, Eliza was furious with me because she got scared watching the movie, and Maddie was upset because Xander's mother wouldn't let him spend the night. Making matters worse, someone had left the screen door open, and every moth in Fort Collins had found its way inside.

"I can't believe this," I told Nat, as one by one, we vacuumed up the moths later that night. At 12, he was the oldest, and I coached his roller hockey team. "Are you guys always this crazy?"

"No way," he said. "We're usually much worse!"

After Nat finally went to bed, I hobbled to the refrigerator. I wasn't a big beer drinker but understood now why Holly had left it for me. When I opened the door and reached in, I found her note.

Molly-

Beer in your cereal will help!

~H

I woke early the next morning to the sound of blaring hip-hop music and looked at the clock. 7:30 a.m. I was already exhausted. "Note to self," I said aloud, "No children."

I made breakfast and took the kids outside, where Nat, Jesse and I could play roller hockey in the street, Maddie could play with Xander and Eliza could do whatever it was that Eliza liked to do, all within my sight. We spent the day in the sunshine, jumping on the trampoline, swimming and staying up late, dancing around the house and making too much noise. I was beginning to rethink my "No Children" clause.

But when I woke Monday morning, still tired, there was a strange pain in my abdomen that felt like a cross between indigestion and PMS. I was sure the kids had just worn me out but decided to break out the water balloons anyway. Our friendly game of toss-the-balloon quickly became a neighborhood-wide water war, complete with buckets, hoses and an oversized slingshot. Kids seemed to be coming from every house, and before I knew it, there were at least 20 of us.

"Hey Nat," I said. We were hiding from Jesse and Maddie in the bushes, both with a water balloon in each hand.

"Yeah?"

"I'm not feeling so hot. I'm going to run into the house for a few minutes. Can you keep an eye on things?"

"Sure. You OK?"

"I'll be fine." I handed him both of my balloons. "Make good use of these."

Inside, I rushed to the bathroom. The pain in my belly had gotten worse since the morning, and I felt like I had to go – *really* go.

I sat down on the toilet, holding onto the steadily worsening pain in the lower right side of my belly and waited for something to happen. I waited and waited, until finally, something ejected itself. That was that.

When the stabbing had subsided some, I stood up and glanced into the porcelain bowl, only to find the water bright red with blood. Terrified, I rushed to the phone to call my doctor. My heart was racing when the nurse finally got on the phone.

"Hi, Miss McMaster. What can I do for you?" she asked calmly.

"Well," I began, realizing how gross this would sound. "I just tried to go to the bathroom but couldn't, and when I got up, there was nothing but blood in the toilet."

"Were you urinating, or trying to have a BM?" I hadn't heard it phrased like that since I'd seen my pediatrician.

"Umm. BM."

"A lot of blood?"

"Well, I guess. Maybe not." I felt embarrassed, realizing that I was probably overreacting.

"Well, don't worry. It's probably just a hemorrhoid, or maybe you wiped too hard. You can make an appointment and we'll see what's going on. Her soothing, confident voice confirmed that I was fine.

"Thanks," I said, relieved that nothing serious was wrong with me. I made an appointment for the following day.

On Tuesday morning, I woke with a dull ache in my belly, not nearly as harsh as the day before, but still an ache. When the kids realized that I still wasn't feeling well, they treated me to eggs and toast in bed. Feeling guilty after I told them that they would have to ride the bus after the long, holiday weekend, I finally crawled out of bed and forced myself into the bathroom, nervous about using the toilet. I was relieved when there was no blood and the pain in my belly seemed to lessen, so I loaded the kids into the car and drove them to school just like I had promised.

When I got back to the house, I felt almost back to normal. "Must have been a 24-four-hour flu bug I caught from those crazy kids," I told Bill the cat. I called Dr. Weston's office and canceled the appointment for later that morning.

4

MORE SYMPTOMS

◆

Late in the fall of 1998, I was skating more than ever. A new director was hired for the local youth hockey program, and with him came the two players he was managing. "Brian's Monkeys," which is how I referred to them, wanted to play professional hockey, and Brian's job was to help get them there. Every night after games and practices, when the ice was empty, Brian would take his protégés to the rink for their workout, and somehow Rocky and I managed to weasel our way onto the ice with them. I had heard rumors that a national women's professional ice hockey league might be starting in the next few years, and I wanted to be ready. Rocky, on the other hand, always trained harder than anyone I knew, even if there was nothing at the end of the tunnel. He didn't have a tryout or a big game. Every game was big to him and he was constantly preparing. "Be uncommon," he used to tell me. Rocky always went one step further than everyone else. One extra bucket of pucks, one extra lap or an extra set of push-ups – just like the extra set he lifted in the weight room. He always wanted to be in top shape and I was following his lead, or at least trying to keep up.

Each night when we got on the ice, Brian put us to work. He was tough. "You missed the net! Give me 20 push-ups!" "Now - do it again!" he would yell.

Brian made us work hardest on the things we were the worst at. For me, it was handling the puck. One night, he took me into the corner alone and dropped a bucket of pucks at my feet. Then he handed me a single puck.

"You've got five minutes to dribble your puck back and forth around all the others. Don't look down. If I catch you looking down, you're doing bear crawls!"

"OK," I said, chuckling. He was strict, but I got a kick out of his coaching style.

"Five minutes," he repeated with his finger right at my nose.

"Don't stop, or you're doing the crawls."

"Yes, Coach," I said smartly and waited until he turned to get on Rocky's case before I started laughing again. I dropped the puck at my feet and looked at the clock at the far wall. It was almost midnight. "Five minutes," I said aloud, and started dribbling back and forth between my skates and all the other pucks.

Split vision was something I was teaching the kids on Nat's roller hockey team. "It's like driving a car," I told them. "You have to watch directly in front of you but also what's down the road a bit."

Remembering the simple lesson for my 12-year-old roller hockey players, I thought about how difficult it really was. I was hitting pucks left and right and hoping that Brian wasn't watching.

Suddenly, I felt an excruciating stab in the lower right side of my abdomen. I dropped my stick and hunched over, grabbing my belly and gasping for air. As the pain lessened, I dropped down on one knee and tried to catch my breath.

"Molly!" Brian shouted from across the ice. "What the hell are you doing?"

"Sorry, Coach. I just got a cramp," I yelled back meekly.

"Cramp, my ass! I told you if you stopped you were giving me bear crawls, so now that's what you're going to do!"

Part of me wanted to laugh at how tough he thought he was, but the other part was thinking about the professional women's league. I picked up my stick, made fists around the shaft with both hands, shoulder-width apart, and got down on both knees. As I did, the pain in my belly came back, but not nearly as bad as before. So, assuming it was just a cramp, I put both fists on the ice, pulled into a plank position and began to crawl, letting my feet drag behind – the dreaded bear crawl. After a few minutes, I stopped. I was exhausted.

"Molly! Get moving!"

"Alright. Alright."

Again, I put my fists to the ice and began to crawl. I had to make it from one end of the ice to the other and back again, and I had only gone halfway. I crawled a few more feet but had to stop again. My belly was throbbing.

"Molly!"

I felt like my father was yelling at me for staying out too late, and through the pain I began to laugh. With my laughter, my eyes began to water. This was what I wanted – what I had asked for. I wanted to be coached by a dictator who screamed, and when I didn't get it right, he would make me do pushups and bear crawls.

I put my fists to the ice one last time and continued to crawl. I was at least 40 feet away from the end of the ice when I heard Brian yell again.

"Let's go, you guys. Get your gear off!" Relief for a brief and shining moment. Practice was over and just in time. My cramps were getting worse. "Meet me outside in five minutes to run the hills!" Brian said.

I let out a disappointed sigh.

Outside, the stinging cold air bit through my sweaty, long sleeved T-shirt and warm-up pants. We stood in a line at the top of the hill: Rocky, me and Brian's two monkeys.

"Alright, you guys. When I blow the whistle, you're going to run down the hill and then back up, five times. When you get to the top after the fifth hill, drop onto your back, keep your legs straight and extended and lift them about six inches off the ground."

Before I could catch my breath, the whistle had blown, and all four of us were on our way down the hill. Rocky, who was getting over strep throat, added extra torture to his workout by running with his hands above his head.

After the fifth time up, we all dropped to the frosty ground and lay on our backs with our feet in the air, moaning. My cramps were beginning to act up again, but I tried to hold my breath and get through it.

"On the whistle, five more hills," Brian yelled.

"This sucks!" one of the monkeys shouted.

"So, you'd like to do six instead? Fine with me!" Again, Brian blew the whistle and we all ran down and back up the hill six times, before collapsing on our backs at the top with our legs extended and our feet off the ground. My cramps were now excruciating.

"I love it!" Rocky yelled in some psychotic voice I had never heard before.

"You want seven this time?" Brian yelled.

"Yes, sir, may I have another?" Rocky yelled back sarcastically.

"Seven it is then!"

"Rocky, I hate you!" I screamed as the whistle blew again.

When we finished seven hills and collapsed again at the top, I could hardly get my feet off the ground. My abdominal muscles were burning, and the cramps were piercing and ripping. I put one foot down.

"Molly! Do that again, and you'll add another thirty seconds for everyone!" Brian yelled.

I quickly put both feet in the air again, but to loosen the pressure on my belly, I tried to bend my knees and lift my feet higher off the ground. Again, the pain became unbearable, and I had to put a foot down.

"Molly! Quit being a pansy! That's another 30 seconds for everyone!"

"Awww, come on, coach!" the smaller monkey yelled.

"Molly, what the hell's your problem?" Rocky shouted. My belly felt like it would tear open at any moment. I didn't know what was wrong with me but realized that I was in worse shape than I thought. Tears began to well in my eyes again, but I couldn't cry in front of them. I'd never hear the end of it. So I stretched my feet into the air and began to count the seconds. After 20, I couldn't hold it anymore and let both feet touch the ground.

"*Molly*! What's your problem?" Coach yelled.

"I'm sorry, Coach. I guess I just need to do more ab work," I said, feeling out of shape and lazy and on the verge of tears.

"Alright, you guys. That's enough for tonight," Brian said. I looked at my watch. It was 1:15 a.m. Finally. I stood up to go home for the night, and in the private darkness in my car, I held onto my belly and let the tears fall.

Classes began the following week, and I was changing my major from English to Exercise Sports Science. It was a big switch and would likely make me a perpetual student, but I didn't care. I wanted to live the rest of my life in Colorado anyway. What did it matter if I was in school for seven years instead of four?

The first prerequisite class was First Aid and CPR, and on my first day, I was surrounded by good looking jocks and tall, blond aerobics instructors, rather than the artsy crowd I'd gotten to know.

"I want you to write me a one-page essay about why you are enrolled in this class," the instructor said. "Right now, pull out your notebooks, rip out a piece of paper and tell me why you are taking First Aid and CPR." I almost laughed. Writing was something I *could* do. I began to write about my dream of being a women's college hockey coach, my current 12-and-under boys' roller hockey team, and how I was changing my major to Exercise and Sports Science with a minor in Coaching. Suddenly, I heard what sounded like a cat when it gets angry, right before the hissing starts.

"Ree-ooo-rrrrrr." Where was that coming from? It started again, but louder and longer this time. "Reeee-oooo-wwww-rr-gggg-rrrr." I looked up from my paper to see the entire class staring at me and realized that the angry cat noise was coming from my stomach. At the same time, the now all too familiar pain in my belly was back. I tried to ignore it and continue writing, but the sound kept coming. "Rrr-eee-ooo-rrr-ggg-rrrrr." I was mortified and clenched my abdominal muscles in hopes that it would stop. Five more minutes of class and then I could go home and hide. Slowly the clock ticked down, but with each passing minute there seemed to be at least four coinciding angry cats.

When the teacher finally dismissed us, I waited until everyone had left before getting up from my seat. That afternoon, I transferred into another class.

5

DR. WESTON

◆

In late October of 1998, the pain in my belly was with me all the time, worse somehow, and yet still bearable, which seemed odd. I remembered it being so excruciating at Holly's when I had spent the weekend with the kids back in July. How could it have possibly gotten worse? I finally decided that I should see a doctor, and for the first time, met my primary care physician in person.

"Hi, Molly," she said as she entered the room. "I'm Dr. Weston."

"Hi," I laughed nervously from the exam table.

"What seems to be the trouble today?" She was soft-spoken and seemed like a laid-back and outdoorsy Colorado girl. I liked her already.

"I've been having really bad stomach pain recently." I gestured toward my belly. "And it makes strange noises sometimes."

"What kind of noises?"

"Weird, growling-type noises," I said.

"Can you show me where it hurts?"

From my position lying on her table, I pointed to the lower right side of my belly, and she began pushing deep into it and then forward, as though kneading dough.

"Well, everything seems OK in there. There's no evidence of obstruction. Does this hurt?"

Her fingers were cold, and although the pressure wasn't comfortable, it didn't exactly hurt. "No," I said. "Not really."

"Molly, when was your last bowel movement?" I jerked slightly at her bluntness.

"I'm not sure," I stumbled. "A few days ago, I guess?"

She lowered my shirt over my belly and helped me sit up on the table.

"I want you to get yourself some Mylanta. I believe you have what is called a spastic colon." I wanted to laugh. I'd heard that I was spastic before, but not my colon. "It's common in women your age. Do you have a heating pad at home?"

"Hot water bottle," I said.

"Good. Use that when it acts up, and take some Mylanta."

"Usually when it hurts, I have a hot bath," I told her.

"That will work too, but try the hot water bottle," she smiled as she reached for the door. "Call me if it doesn't work."

"Thanks, Dr. Weston." Spastic colon. Common for my age. That was easy enough. I was feeling better already.

However, the following week, the pain was worse, so I called Dr. Weston's office and made another appointment.

"Hi Molly," she said. "How are you?"

"Not so good," I said. "I've been throwing up, and the pain in my stomach has gotten worse." She laid me down on the table, lifted my shirt and began kneading again with chilly fingertips.

"Can you describe the pain for me?"

"It's pretty much a constant ache, but every now and then there's a sharp pain, right about here," I said, pointing to the lower right side of my belly again.

"And how long does the sharp pain last?"

"Probably 30 or 40 seconds," I guessed, "and then it goes back to the dull pain for about a minute, until the sharper pain starts again. I'm having trouble sleeping at night because of it."

She unwrapped a needle and prepped my arm to draw some blood.

"I still think it's a colonic spasm, or maybe Irritable Bowel Syndrome, which is also very common in young women."

I cringed and looked away as she pushed the needle into my arm.

"I'm going to do a CBC, and I'm also going to send you in for an X-ray to rule out anything more serious."

I didn't have any idea what the CBC was all about, but her confidence was soothing, and my pain was lessened while I was in her office.

"OK," I said.

"My nurse will be here in a few minutes to give you an appointment for the X-ray."

"Thanks," I said.

She left the room.

The next morning, I arrived at the hospital and cursed myself for not putting on makeup before leaving the house. The X-ray tech was tall, good-looking and not much older than me.

"Hi Molly," he said, as though we were old friends. "How is the pain today?"

"Better," I said.

"Can you tell me when your last bowel movement was?"

I nearly choked. I hardly knew this guy and he was already asking about my bowel movements. It had been bad enough having to tell Dr. Weston, and I could feel my face getting warmer. "Um, I guess it was this morning," I said, remembering something jagged and paper-thin.

"Good. Thanks."

"Thank *you*," I said under my breath while I followed him through the stark and overly lit hallway and into a darkened X-ray room. I was no longer worried about my lack of makeup.

The following morning, the phone rang.

"Hi, Molly. This is Jill, Dr. Weston's nurse."

"Hi Jill."

"I just wanted to let you know that your blood test came back normal."

"Thanks. I'm feeling a bit better too," I said.

"Your white count was a bit high, but that's really nothing to worry about. You're probably just fighting something off."

"Good," I said, happy to know that I would be OK.

"Your X-ray did show a significant amount of retained stool though, and Dr. Weston feels that you're just constipated," she continued. "She would like you to try some suppositories."

You've got to be kidding.

"You can pick them up at any pharmacy."

"OK. Thanks, Jill," I said. Something about the word "suppositories" made me want to hurry off the phone.

We hung up and I forced myself to make the trip to the drugstore. I picked up things I needed around the house, and some that I didn't, and finally worked my way to the pharmacist's counter.

"Can I pay for all of these here?" I asked.

"Sure," he said and began to ring me up.

"Um, I need to get one more thing though. My father sent me to the store for suppositories. Can you tell me where those would be?

"Sure. They're right over there at the beginning of aisle three."

"Thanks," I said. "Or should I say, my father thanks you?" I smiled unconvincingly and was sure I heard him say, "Yeah, right," as I turned away.

By early November, four months after it started, the pain in my belly seemed to have weakened. I had been hired at the brand-new ice rink in Windsor, about 10 minutes south of Fort Collins, as an ice-skating instructor, youth hockey coach and --- most exciting --- Zamboni driver. We were aiming for a Christmas-week opening, but until the building was complete, I hauled dirt into the facility and helped install the ice. It was manual labor, which I loved so much that I strongly considered not going home for Thanksgiving. Unfortunately, Mom and Dad weren't having it.

When I arrived in New York and Mom mentioned that I looked like I had lost some weight, I rushed upstairs to try on some of my old high school clothes. It had become somewhat of a ritual every time I visited my parents, but this time I could get everything on for the first time since my senior year. I was ecstatic and silently credited my workouts for finally paying off.

My visit was off to a great start, but halfway through the week my nearly forgotten abdominal pain was back and seemed worse than ever. Still going on Dr. Weston's assumption that I was constipated, I went to the grocery store and awkwardly read pill boxes and medicine bottles until I found a green glass bottle of lemon-flavored Phospho soda that promised to do the trick. I hated liquid medicines, but I knew that I had to hold it down for my own good.

When I got home, I took the bottle into the shower and made up a game. I washed my face and then took a huge swig, cringing at the taste. Then I washed my hair and took another large gulp, nearly gagging. On and on the game went until the liquid in the bottle was gone. Then, I waited.

After about an hour, my belly began to gurgle, and then after two hours it felt as if it was at war with itself. I made a trip to the bathroom, and then another and another. I never left the house that night, and never went farther than 20 feet from the bathroom, but the pain and pressure finally seemed to be subsiding.

On Thursday, I sat across the large dining room table from Rob and his new girlfriend Aimee for our annual Thanksgiving dinner. I knew she was a nurse, but didn't want to talk about poop with her any more than I had wanted to talk about it with Dr. Weston or the cute X-ray tech. Besides, my belly felt less full thanks to the Phospho soda I'd forced myself to drink the day before. Still, my appetite was virtually nonexistent, and for the first

Thanksgiving ever, I only sampled a few of the items on the table. Even the mashed potatoes --- my favorite --- didn't look very appealing, and I only had one small bite of apple pie.

"What? Are you *dieting*?" my brother asked.

"No," I snapped, "just not very hungry."

"Would you rather she ate like the rest of us?" his girlfriend Aimee laughed, pointing around the table at the overflowing plates.

I was grateful that she had diverted the attention from me and wished I was more comfortable talking with her about my belly trouble. On Thanksgiving, I would normally overeat just like everyone else, but now the dull ache was a constant in my life and my appetite was disappearing. I didn't know what was wrong, but my old clothes were fitting again and I wasn't going to complain.

Back in Colorado, nothing changed. I still wasn't hungry and almost found it convenient not having to bring lunch to work. A chocolate milkshake doubled as an entire day's worth of food. That was working out just fine, until the day I had to call in sick.

"Hello?"

"Dan?" I asked.

"Yes."

"It's Molly."

"Oh, hey, Moll. Geez. I hardly recognized your voice. You sound horrible. You OK?"

"Actually, no. I'm not going to be able to make it into work today," I mumbled. "I don't know what's wrong with me, but my stomach is killing me."

"OK. Get better soon, and just call me when you're ready to come back to work."

"Thanks, Dan," I said.

Then I punched my parents' number into the cordless phone.

"Hello?"

"Mom?"

"Molly? Are you OK? You sound terrible."

"Mom," I managed to say, still mumbling. "I can't get out of bed, and I've been throwing up all morning."

"Oh, gosh, Molly. Did you call your doctor?"

"No. She hasn't been able to help me. She says I'm just constipated. My stomach hurts so badly." I was crying and held the phone tightly against my cheek, my face buried in a pillow.

"Mom, please make the pain go away," I begged.

"Molly. Stay there. I'm going to call your doctor."

"She won't be able to help me," I cried.

"I'll call you back," she said.

I put the phone down and let my eyelids fall.

"Hello?" I clasped the phone tightly between clammy fingers.

"Hi, Molly?"

"Yes?" I rubbed my swollen eyes and looked at the clock. 11:30 a.m.

"This is Jill, from Dr. Weston's office."

"Hi." I cleared my throat and tried to sound awake.

"Your Mom called from New York. She said you're still not feeling well. What seems to be the trouble?"

"Um, well. I've been throwing up all morning. I can't hold any food down." I sounded like a five-year-old child who had just scraped her knee and wanted to be held by her mommy.

"The constipation is getting pretty bad, huh?"

"I guess so," I croaked again softly. "I haven't been able to get out of bed. I can't even hold any water down

44

and …" I stopped and took a breath before continuing. "I have a horrible pain in my stomach." My voice was rising in pitch and tears were spattering my face. "I can't even get out of bed," I repeated.

"OK, Molly. Breathe for a minute." I quieted down but still found myself gasping for breath. "If I call in a prescription, could you go pick it up?"

"I can't even get out of bed," I repeated.

"Alright then, we'll have to use a pharmacy that delivers. I'm going to order you a prescription of Lactulose. It will help to loosen you up and should clear this up in a few hours."

"Thank you." I was relieved to hear that something could be sent to the house.

I put the phone down and let my body soar away again, to a place where nothing hurt, until the next wave of pain pulled me back. I slept on and off like that for the next few hours, grasping at what sleep I could get.

The impatient ringing of the doorbell finally woke me, and I struggled to pull myself up from bed. A pimply teen-age boy stood in the doorway holding a white paper bag. I must have looked horrendous, but I didn't even care. All I wanted was for the pain to go away.

I limped down the hall and into the kitchen. The room was tilting slightly. All I needed was to take the medicine and go back to bed. I could sleep through it, and in a few hours everything would be better.

I nearly gagged when I saw that Lactulose was a liquid. Again, I would have to force myself to drink it. For a moment, I remembered Mom and Dad chasing me around the house when I was home sick from elementary school and holding me down on the kitchen counter to give me a teaspoon of cough syrup. They had triumphantly tilted the spoon back, only to see, within seconds, a spray of grape-flavored stickiness all over the cabinets. This time I had to do it on my own.

I opened the refrigerator, reached for a bottle of ginger ale and poured myself a glass of the bubbly gold liquid. Then, I fumbled through the silverware drawer and found the biggest spoon. I grabbed a roll of paper towels, just in case.

I put everything on a tray and slowly dragged myself back into my bedroom, then placed the tray on the bed next to my puke bowl and carefully sat down so as not to tip anything over. All the activity had taken everything out of me. I lay back and closed my eyes, wishing everything would just get better on its own, like a scraped knee. You could leave it alone and eventually, it would heal. What was wrong with me?

Another stabbing pain in my abdomen forced me to sit up again. Feeling as though I were drunk, I gripped the top of the brown glass bottle, twisted it and broke the seal. The grossly sweet odor of the liquid penetrated my nostrils and I nearly dropped the bottle. I poured the thick, clear syrup into the spoon and willed myself to keep it down. I gulped it, gagging at its harsh taste and texture. Then I snatched my ginger ale chaser, guzzling as much as I could, but couldn't rid the taste. I lay back down but within a few minutes began to feel the medicine rising in the back of my throat. I sat up, grabbed the bowl and heaved a few times.

My plan was to wait for the queasiness to pass before making a second attempt at holding down the foul liquid, but again my body rejected it.

After a third attempt and an hour and a half of tears and frustration at not being able to relieve the pain, I called Dr. Weston's office again.

"After hours." The woman who answered obviously had better things to do with her time.

"I'm trying to reach Dr. Weston," I begged, sounding not unlike someone who had been lying face down in her pillow and crying.

"She's gone home for the day. Is this an emergency?"

"Well, yes. Umm, no." I couldn't decide. Was it an emergency?

"I really need to speak with someone. Is there a nurse there please?" I sniffed.

"Let me take your name and I'll page the nurse on call. She'll call you back within a half hour."

"OK. Thanks." I closed my eyes and wished for the pain to go away and got the next best thing. I fell asleep.

When I woke to the sound of ringing, it was dark. My eyes found the glowing green of the clock and I read 8:36 p.m. The ache in my belly was still there. Why the hell hadn't that nurse called me back?

"Hello?"

"Molly McMaster," she announced. I hated answering the phone and being told who I was, rather than asked. "This is Theresa. I'm the nurse on call tonight."

What time did I call the office? It must have been at least two hours earlier. I felt another stab in my belly, but I would forgive her. There must have been a good excuse.

"What seems to be the problem, Miss McMaster? It says here that you're constipated."

"Um, yeah. Dr. Weston had some Lactulose sent over to me earlier today, and I've been trying to keep it down all afternoon but can't."

"What do you mean, you *can't?*" she asked. She made it sound like I hadn't handed in a homework assignment.

"I mean I've taken it three times and thrown it back up every time. I think something else may be wrong with me. My belly *really* hurts."

"I'm sorry to hear that, but if you want to get better, you *need* to keep the Lactulose down!"

Why was she treating me like I'd just spit up my Flintstones on purpose? I felt my face getting hot again as I tried to control my temper and hold back tears. How was I supposed to keep it down if I kept throwing it up?

I took a deep breath and let it out slowly, hoping to ease both my pain and my frustration. "I understand that I'm supposed to take the medicine," I began calmly, "but I *really* think that something else may be wrong with me."

"*Miss McMaster*, you're constipated. You need to keep the medicine down!" she repeated.

"I understand that, but I haven't been able to, and I'm not someone who throws up regularly! This has been going on for the past few days!"

I felt bad to have bothered her but stopped short when I realized that I was about to apologize. What was I thinking? She was supposed to be helping me. Instead, I felt like a burden. I was sick of being calm and nice.

"*Miss* McMaster," she began, but I quickly took advantage of my anger and shut her down.

"I *know* I need to keep it down!" I snapped, "But I can't! I can't control whether my body keeps something inside it or not! What the hell else am I supposed to do?"

Silence.

Was she still there? For a brief moment, I was embarrassed for reacting the way that I had, until she spoke again.

"*Miss* McMaster. First of all, you *need* to calm down!" she said sternly. I pictured myself reaching through the phone and grabbing her tightly by the throat, forcing every last bit of breath out of her lifeless body. I saw her face turning a brilliant reddish-blue, and she couldn't speak. I wanted her to feel just a portion of the pain that I was feeling.

"I suggest that you try digitally stimulating your bowels," she said.

"*Excuse me?*" I couldn't believe what I just heard.

"It says in your records that Dr. Weston already prescribed suppositories and you called her back and said that wasn't working. Since you *won't* hold down the Lactulose, I suggest that you digitally stimulate your bowels."

I was confused. I didn't remember telling her that I *wouldn't* hold the medicine down.

"And what, *exactly*, do you mean by that?" I asked smartly.

"You need to insert your finger…" she began.

"You know what, Theresa?" I interrupted. "Never mind! You aren't helping me anyway!" With tears of pain and frustration, I slammed down the phone.

When I woke the next day in my warm bed, I didn't want to move, I didn't want to speak. The sharp pain was unbearable. I had no energy and couldn't do anything to help myself.

Finally, I counted to three and forced myself to reach for the phone. It took everything I had just to punch the numbers into the phone. I heard a ring and then a second one. Click. Thank God! "Hello. You have reached the McMaster's. We can't come to the phone right now…" Shit! I waited for the beep and tried to speak, but all I could choke out was barely a whisper. "Mom? Where are you? Please call me." Click.

I hung up the phone and closed my eyes.

I was jerked awake by another jab of pain. The cordless phone was resting on the pillow beside me. I put my fingers around it and willed myself out of the bed. The pain was piercing and horrible, as though I'd been kicked hard in the belly with a soccer cleat.

Slowly I punched the buttons and again waited through the ringing, tears collecting on my cheeks.

"Hello? Dr. Weston's office. May I help you?" I pictured a thirty-something mother of two with a strawberry blonde bob.

"I need to speak with Dr. Weston, please."

"Please hold." I was so sick of holding.

"Hello? How may I help you?" It was a new voice, but it wasn't Dr. Weston.

"I need to speak with Dr. Weston, please," I repeated irritably.

"She's with a patient right now. I'm her nurse, Jill. Can I help you?"

"This is Molly McMaster. I've called several times."

"Oh. Hi, Molly. I'm the nurse who ordered the Lactulose for you last night. How are you feeling?"

"I'm still having severe pain. I can't walk, and I haven't been able to eat or drink anything in three days, including the Lactulose. I just threw up a glass of water!"

"Can you come to see Dr. Weston today?"

"I can try," I said.

"We'll be here waiting for you. Come in whenever you can."

"Thanks," I said, a bit annoyed that she hadn't been more help.

I hung up the phone and lay back down, gritting my teeth as the pain passed through my belly.

After a few minutes and a few more belly pains had come and gone, I made myself stand again. I slid into my blue warm-up pants, the closest thing I could find, and slowly put a sweatshirt over the T-shirt that I'd been wearing for the past three days. I covered my unwashed, matted hair with a black Colorado Avalanche baseball cap. Then I sat back down, took a breath, and reached for my sneakers, pushing myself to finish getting dressed so I could lay back down and rest. Catching a glimpse of myself in a mirror, I managed a small smile. I was a mess. I hadn't showered in days or even brushed my hair. The funny part was that I couldn't have cared less. All I wanted was for the pain to go away.

I drove slowly and carefully, grimacing when I hit a rut or pothole in the road. The pain was excruciating, and the 15-minute drive seemed like hours. When I had finally arrived and was safely inside, I told the receptionist I was there and took a seat.

Twenty minutes passed. What could they be doing in there that was so important? I thought to myself. Why couldn't they move me somewhere where I could lay down?

Finally, my name was called. I was ushered into a small room and seated on the crinkly, paper-covered examining table.

"OK, Molly, what can we do for you today?" the nurse asked.

I tried to control my tears.

"I can't eat or drink. I'm tired and I'm weak, and my belly is *killing* me." I was angry that I had to explain again.

"When was the last time you held any food down?"

"Three days ago."

"Hmmm. Let's see what Dr. Weston thinks." She disappeared and I was left alone to survey the light pink room, which reeked of disinfectant. I was staring at a poster about human reproduction when Dr. Weston finally waltzed through the door. The calm demeanor from my previous visits now looked like terrible boredom.

"So, you're still having abdominal pain, huh, Molly?"

"Yes," I said, irritated that I was going through this yet again.

"And you haven't been able to eat?"

"No."

"What's the pain in your abdomen like? Is it constant?" she asked. Hadn't I already been through this with her?

I sighed. "Yes, it's constant. But every few minutes it gets extremely sharp, like someone is stabbing me from the inside."

"And how long does the sharp pain last?" she asked, jotting notes on my chart.

"About 45 seconds, and then it goes back to normal." *Normal.* I couldn't believe I had just used that word. Did I even know what normal was anymore?

"We already did the X-rays, and they came back negative for a blockage," the doctor said, "but I guess we should order some again to rule out anything more serious."

"I haven't been able to keep any food or liquids down," I said, choking up with tears. I was practically pleading for her to make the hurting stop.

"Molly. I really don't know why you're crying. You're *just* constipated."

My heart sank, and in that moment, my fear and naivete turned into vicious anger. I wanted to slap her condescending face.

"We're going to do a pelvic and rectal exam now too, just to be sure. Do you want some ginger ale first to settle your stomach?"

"I *told* you, I haven't been able to keep anything down," I snapped.

"We'll give you a shot of Compazine. It's a muscle relaxer and it will let you keep things down."

"Fine," I said.

She swabbed alcohol on my arm. This time, when compared to the stabbing pain in my belly, the needle felt like a tickle. In a few moments, the pain weakened. The nurse returned with a red plastic cup, fizzing with icy ginger ale. I sipped it and then sat back on the examining table, seething with anger.

The next morning, I woke to pain that was slightly dulled.

The phone rang.

"Hi, Molly? This is Dr. Weston. How are you feeling?"

"A little bit better," I answered.

"We got the results back from your X-rays yesterday. I looked them over myself and everything seems to be normal, except there is still a substantial amount of stool built up in the large intestine. There's no evidence of obstruction though, and that's what I was after. I want you to keep drinking a lot of fluids and take some Milk of Magnesia. Try some FiberCon too."

"OK," I said. Didn't I see a TV commercial for Fiber Con? A bunch of old people were running in a meadow, if I remembered correctly.

"Call me if you have any more trouble."

I was disappointed that the diagnosis hadn't changed but because I was feeling mildly better, I was hopeful that my body was beginning to finally heal itself. If it was truly just constipation, the only thing I could do was exactly what she said. Certainly I would feel better by Christmas.

6

WINTER

◆

As the Colorado plains turned from lush green to dull brown, and the Rockies became capped with snow, I found myself spending more and more time at the new rink. The grand opening was set for a few days before Christmas, and to stay on schedule, I drove in a blustery snowstorm and worked all night helping to flood the rink with water from an old fire hose. We sprayed a layer of water and then waited an hour while the compressors did their job. Once the first layer was frozen, we sprayed another coating of water and waited another hour. On and on it went through the night and I loved it. The paycheck was just an added bonus. But as the holidays neared, and everything around me seemed so hopeful, my optimism dimmed because of the pain in my belly. I began to believe that my tolerance for pain was increasing as well. I flew home to New York for Christmas and did my best to pretend everything was fine.

When I tried on my old clothes again at Mom and Dad's, I couldn't believe my eyes. The pants that I hadn't been able to get over my hips six months ago, and were snug a month ago at Thanksgiving, were now actually loose. I turned my body from side to side in front of the mirror in my old bedroom, admiring my figure. Even with the odd bulge below my belly, I was thinner than I had been in years. I had no idea what I'd done, but I was thrilled.

Each time I ran into an old friend that week, my ego swelled as I heard the same compliments over and over again. By the time I flew back to Colorado, I had ditched my baggy sweatshirts and warm-up pants and instead packed most of my high school clothes, ready to introduce the new me.

I landed in Colorado the day before New Year's Eve and felt the same slight belly pain I'd been having all week. I brushed it off once again, praying that the stabbing pains weren't coming back, but the next morning, I awoke with a puncturing sensation tearing through my abdomen. I didn't want to miss the New Year's Eve party I'd been invited to, so I took four Advil and spent the day going back and forth between a hot bath and the couch, trying to will the pain away. By six o'clock, when the pain had not subsided and I was exhausted from fighting it, I heated up my hot water bottle, climbed into my bed and pulled up the covers. Certainly I would wake up with plenty of time to shower and head out.

"What a Lame-O I am," I said aloud as I closed my eyes. How could I possibly be curled up in bed at home instead of arriving early at the party to greet the CSU Men's Ice Hockey Team? I gritted my teeth as another slow stab pierced my belly and then fell asleep.

My eyes opened sharply in the dark, and it wasn't until the second ring that I realized where I was. I crawled out of bed, dizzy with confusion and snatched the receiver from the desk.

"Hello?"

"What the hell are you doing home?"

My friend Chuck's voice shot through me but couldn't pull me entirely from my dazed state of consciousness.

"What?" I looked at the clock. 11:45. Was it morning or night?

"I called to leave the last message of the year on your machine!" Music and laughter vibrated through the phone as I began to focus. "Why aren't you out celebrating?" Chuck asked.

"Oh, man!" I yelled into the receiver. "I've slept through half the party! Happy New Year!"

"Are you OK?" Chuck asked.

"Uh, yeah. I just laid down for a quick catnap, but that was almost six hours ago! I have to go! I'll call you tomorrow!"

I threw the phone down and grabbed the closest pair of jeans, slipping them on as I ran into the bathroom. Then I smeared on some lipstick and ran a brush through my hair before pulling it into a tight ponytail. Everyone would probably already be drunk anyway, I reasoned before running out the front door.

I got in the car, put the gas to the floor and arrived at the party with just enough time to grab a drink and start the countdown to the New Year. I told myself I would only stay long enough for one drink and then head home, but one drink turned into two and two into four. The buzz seemed to help the pain in my belly and eventually I fell asleep on the couch. I dreamed of a wonderful 1999 with no pain, unaware that the worst pain was still to come.

The first week in January started gently and I considered that maybe my body really was finally trying to heal itself. I had taken the semester off from school to save some money and train for a spring tryout with a women's AAA hockey team in Ottawa.

The rink was finished, and I loved my job driving the Zamboni, coaching youth hockey and teaching ice skating lessons. I'd been invited to play in the Men's Competitive Hockey League, the top league in the area, and would be the first woman to do so. I even bought a plane ticket to Daytona Beach for our family trip in February, when we would visit with my brother and celebrate my twenty-third birthday. Except for the stupid pain in my belly, life seemed perfect, until one by one, the threads began to unravel.

The constant dull ache on the lower right side of my abdomen was back, constant and sharp, instead of intermittent. My appetite was almost nonexistent. I was throwing up. Then there was the exhaustion. I tried to push myself to work out and play hockey, but most days I had trouble getting out of bed. I called in sick a few times, and on my days off I stayed in bed or camped out on the couch in front of the television, not wanting to move or even breathe too deeply for fear that I would make the pain worse. After the fourth time I called in sick, my boss told me I wasn't dependable and not to come back. My heart shattered.

January had no mercy and I finally admitted defeat. There was nothing left for me in Colorado. Something was seriously wrong inside me and I knew that I needed my family. I talked it over with Mom and Dad and we decided that I would move back home to New York in a few weeks.

On February 2, 1999, I went to Dr. Weston's office for the last time, nauseated and with unbelievable pain in my bloated abdomen. I couldn't button the top button of my jeans, yet my clothes were looser than ever.

"I haven't eaten anything in *two* days," I pleaded.

But she stayed true to her original diagnosis and gave me another shot of Compazine.

"Drink lots of fluids," she said, but this time, Dr. Weston *finally* referred me to a gastroenterologist at the local hospital.

I sat in the waiting room of the GI Center in the dank basement of the Poudre Valley Hospital filled with dread. I clutched my belly with my left hand and a pen with my right, pondering what my future held. I knew what GI stood for. There would be no X-rays this time around.

"Do you have any questions for the doctor today?" was the final question on the clipboard on my lap.

"What's wrong with me???" I scrawled.

I looked at the clock. Over 45 minutes had passed. What were they doing?

"Molly McMaster?" the nurse finally called, glancing around the room at the patients. She seemed surprised when I stood up, as I was the youngest in the room by 50 years.

I followed her down the brightly lit corridor, which was much less intimidating than I had assumed, with its paintings of mountains and flowers on the walls.

In the small examining room, I was alone again. The fear began to rise from my feet, as if I was walking on hot coals.

Suddenly, the door flew open. "Miss McMaster," the doctor announced. "I'm Dr. Graves."

"Hi."

"I understand you're having some constipation."

Right to the point. I gulped at his straight-forwardness. "Um, yeah."

"When was your last bowel movement?"

Couldn't he have started with some of the less embarrassing questions? "The other day, I think." I wanted to sink deep into the exam table.

"I'm going to do a quick exam, so if you'd put this on." He handed me a large blue paper gown. "I'll be back in just a few minutes."

"OK," I croaked.

"Jeans off. Underwear can stay on," he said, as he closed the door behind him.

The fear was overwhelming. I glanced around the room and a dark object caught my eye. What the *hell* was that thing? It looked like a shiny, black patent-leather snake, standing straight up from the floor, about three feet, before twisting and curving like a pretzel. Where was he going to stick that? I removed my jeans and wrapped myself in the blue paper gown. Just as I finished, there was a knock on the door. I didn't even have time to answer before Dr. Graves walked right in.

"Are you all set then?"

"Yup," I said, trying to hide my fear.

"OK, good. What seems to be the trouble today, Miss McMaster?"

"My belly really hurts." I sounded like I was five years old and immediately regretted my choice of words, but quickly went on hoping that he didn't notice. "I'm nauseated and I've been throwing up a lot."

"How's your appetite?"

"Not so good. I've lost a lot of weight over the past three or four months." I didn't let on that I'd been rather excited about that.

"Has there been any blood or mucus in your stool lately?"

"No." Not lately, anyway, I thought to myself.

"What about stress?"

"What do you mean?" I asked.

"Have you been under any stress lately? Your job? School? Friends? Boyfriend?"

"Oh. No. Not really. Well, I did just get fired from my job and will be leaving next week to move back to New York." That didn't seem stressful when compared with the pain I'd been enduring for months.

"OK. Would you please lie down on your back on the examination table?"

I shuffled across the paper, inching back on the table and laid my head on the pillow. My blue paper dress crinkled as his clammy fingers pressed my belly.

"Does this hurt?"

"Um, a little bit," I answered, gritting my teeth.

"How about this?" His fingers maneuvered their way across my belly as if he was playing a baby grand.

"Mmm, hmm," I answered.

"Could you roll over onto your belly for me?"

When I was on my stomach, the familiar and embarrassing 'cat screeching' started as his cold fingers played Mozart over my kidneys. The pain was increasing as Dr. Graves finally spoke again.

"OK. You can sit up now."

Holding my gown closed, I wondered why there wasn't a female nurse in the room with the doctor.

Dr. Graves scribbled on his prescription pad.

"I think Dr. Weston was right on with the constipation, and I'm going to go a little bit further and say that you've got Irritable Bowel Syndrome. That means that your bowels aren't working exactly as they're supposed to. It's probably stress-related since you've just recently lost your job and will be moving. I'm going to prescribe Metamucil in the morning, one heaping spoonful. Drink lots of water during the day and take two FiberCon at night. Go ahead and make the move to New York, and if this hasn't regulated itself by the time you get there you might want to follow up with your primary care physician."

Then he was gone. It amazed me that I was with the doctor for only 10 minutes. But I didn't care. The only thing that mattered was that the scary patent-leather snake never made an appearance.

The day before I planned to leave for New York, I took a long hot bath to drown my belly pain before putting on a pair of my high school jeans, a cream-colored sweater set and boots. The jeans were loose, but I had to leave the top button undone.

At seven o'clock, I left the house to meet Rocky and a few of his military friends who were celebrating his 26th birthday. I wasn't hungry and hadn't had an appetite in days, but I didn't want to miss my last opportunity to see him before I left Colorado.

When I arrived, they were already at the bar, waiting for a table.

"Hey, Moll! Ya want a drink?" Rocky asked when he saw me.

"No thanks, Rock. Happy birthday though." I managed a smile as I gave him a hug. I definitely didn't feel like having a drink.

"No drink?"

"No, thanks."

When we were finally seated at a table, I forced myself to order *something* and decided I could nibble on a chicken Caesar salad. I couldn't believe that I had become one of those girls who ordered salad and water for dinner.

"You OK, Moll?" Rocky asked. "You're never this quiet!"

I was exhausted and hurting and wanted to go home and fall asleep in another hot bath. That was the only place I could find any relief from the pain. But instead, not knowing when I would see Rocky again, I listened to the jokes and laughter as if I was watching a sitcom and I tried desperately not to cry. Finally, I couldn't stand it any longer.

"Rock, I'm not feeling so well. And I really don't want to ruin your birthday. I think I'm just going to head home."

"Ya sure, Kid?"

I nodded my head. "I'm sure," I said.

"Alright, I'll walk ya out."

We pushed through the sea of people and out the front door.

"I'll miss you," I told Rocky when we got to my car.

"You'll be back," he said. I'm sure he thought it was what I wanted to hear, but in the back of my mind I didn't believe I would ever come back to this place I had finally begun to call home

I threw my arms around Rocky, hiding my face so he wouldn't see the tears welling up in my eyes. "I really am going to miss you."

"I'll miss ya too, Kid," he said. "Are you crying?" he asked. "There's no *crying* in baseball," he joked, throwing me one of Tom Hanks' lines from the movie *A League of Their Own*.

I giggled through my tears. Rocky's ability to make me laugh no matter what was one of his greatest features.

"Seriously, Moll, don't cry. I'll see ya again soon."

We would be friends for a long time to come, that much I knew, but I didn't have the heart to tell him that the tears were not for him, but about the horrific pain in my body.

"Call me," I said. I closed the car door and drove away before I allowed myself to sob. I wanted to rip my own stomach out. Why couldn't anyone figure out what was wrong?

When I was safe at home, I drew a hot bath and sat on the floor next to the tub, still crying.

"I won't be surprised if you're back here within a year."

Christian's words echoed in my ears as though he were sitting next to me on the cold tile. I had lived in Colorado for three and a half years, much longer than he had predicted, but I was returning to New York in a few short days. I felt like a failure. I couldn't handle a little pain in my belly and had to run home to Mommy and Daddy. I sat on the floor with my head against the tub and cried, hating Christian at that moment with every piece of my soul.

My head began to spin and throb, forcing me to lie down on the cold tiled floor. Suddenly, and without warning, I felt my stomach turn. I quickly sat up and grabbed the toilet just in time to throw up undigested chicken Caesar salad and a *lot* of water.

7

GOING HOME

◆

The next morning, I slowly packed what remained of my bedroom. I loved living in that house. It was new and in a nice neighborhood, and I had a cute little window seat in my room. I would miss Colorado, but I'd been dealt a hand that I couldn't successfully play on my own. I had to go home.

I slipped my clothes off the hangers and stuffed them into my suitcase, then hauled it outside and crammed it into the midnight blue Saturn. When I went back inside, I collapsed, for the fourth time, in a heap of exhaustion on the now naked mattress. Where had all my energy gone? I lay on the bed for 20 minutes, catching my breath and willing myself to get back up and figure out how to fit the remaining bits of four years of my life into an already overstuffed car.

When it was time to say goodbye, I drove to the rink to watch my women's team practice. Normally I would have wanted nothing more than to suit up and get on the ice with them one last time, but I had finally given in to the pain. I had tried so hard to keep skating, even playing in a game in Denver just a few days before. In the locker room after the game, the pain was so visibly excruciating that one of my teammates asked if I needed to go to the emergency room. That was the moment that something in me finally clicked. I needed help. I had to make it home to New York.

I watched the Flames run my favorite center ice curl drill. I watched them skate, pass and shoot, and for the first time since I'd picked up a hockey stick, I didn't even really care. My passion for hockey was gone. My passion for a lot of things was gone. I wasn't even worried about missing my friends and teammates. I just wanted to say goodbye and get back to New York --- back to where Mom would make everything OK.

My goodbyes were a blur, and then I found myself alone in my car speeding toward Denver and thinking about how easy it would be to turn around and go back and go to sleep. Instead, I fought to keep going. There were roughly 2,000 miles of road ahead of me, yet at mile 38 I was already nodding off.

Somewhere just outside of the Denver city limits, I pulled into a hotel parking lot, turned the car off, and fell asleep within minutes. I had been driving for just over an hour.

The next three days were more of the same. I drove an hour, slept an hour. Then I drove two and slept two. As someone who normally had so much energy, I couldn't understand what was going on. And the pain in my belly was growing sharper and more consuming.

After nearly two full days of driving and sleeping in my car, I stopped at my grandmother's house near Columbus, Ohio, hoping for some decent rest.

"Are you hungry?" she asked as soon as I arrived.

"Not really, Grandma," I told her.

"Let me fix you something to eat," she said. Grandma was intent on feeding me and began bustling in the kitchen.

"Just soup broth please," I begged and then escaped for a hot shower.

When I emerged feeling slightly better, or at least cleaner, she sat me down at the kitchen table with a bowl of chicken noodle soup.

"I added extra noodles," Grandma said. I shuddered at the thought of anything solid going into my belly.

"Is this homemade?" I asked, sipping only the broth.

"Of course. Molly, you really need to eat."

"Grandma, I know," I pleaded, "but I can't."

I sipped as many spoonfuls as I could, which was barely a noticeable amount. "I'm sorry. It's delicious. I don't really have much of an appetite."

We cleaned up the kitchen together and then visited on the couch, and for the first time, I realized that I was enjoying our conversation. She was different one-on-one and seemed interested in what I had been doing with my life. The irony was painful. I finally *wanted* to sit and talk with Grandma, but the consistent stabbing pains wouldn't allow me to focus. Instead, I concentrated on the minute hand on the old grandfather clock in the hallway. Bedtime couldn't come soon enough.

"You should stay a few days and let me show you around town," Grandma said. She seemed genuinely happy to have me there and I felt sorry for her obvious loneliness.

I held my belly as I walked toward the guest room feeling guilty that I had only visited her once before, but I had to get home. Home was the only place where I believed I would find relief from my ever-growing pain.

"I'm so sorry, Grandma," was all that I could say. "I *have* to get home."

In the morning, she made bacon, eggs and toast.

"You need to eat," she said. But she didn't understand.

"I can't." There was nothing else to say. I drank water.

After breakfast, I hugged and kissed Grandma and began the last 12 hours of my hellish ride home.

More than 2,000 miles after my journey had begun, I finally took the left hand turn down Garrison Road and felt the unrelenting jab in the right side of my abdomen. I waited for it to pass and glanced at the clock. It was 11:20 p.m. I felt the stress leaving my body with the reality that in a few minutes I was going to be home with Mom and Dad. Three days of surviving on only water, Gatorade, half a Twinkie and some soup broth at Grandma's were coming to an end. I couldn't remember the last full meal I'd eaten. It must have been the chicken Caesar salad on Rocky's birthday, but that didn't count because I threw it up. It didn't matter. I wasn't hungry ... just *so* damned tired.

I pulled into the driveway, turned the key off and waited for the next pain to pass before sliding out of the car. I could barely lift my legs to climb the two steps to the front door, but felt relief when Mom appeared. For just a second, all the pain left me, and I knew I would be OK.

"Welcome home!" she shrieked. She gave me a bear hug, but I just wanted to lie down with a cool, wet cloth on my forehead and Mom's fingers running through my hair.

"Hi, Mom," I said hoarsely, gripping her and gritting my teeth as I waited for the pain to stop.

Mom put her hand on my forehead. "You don't look well at all," she said. Mom knew I wasn't feeling well over the past months, but she was unprepared for the reality that stood in the doorway.

"You're gray. Let me fix you something to eat. Are you hungry?"

I wasn't, but I knew I needed some kind of energy. "Just soup, please," I said.

"Hi, Mokins," Dad said from around the corner, wearing his familiar old blue robe.

"How are you feeling?" he asked, hugging me.

"OK, I guess," I lied.

Dad went back to bed, and in the kitchen, Mom and I made small talk about my trip.

Within minutes, a steaming mug of chicken noodle soup was in front of me. I had to force down a few spoonfuls. I just wanted to lie down and have all the pain in my belly disappear. I just wanted to sleep – *forever*.

"How was the drive?" she asked.

"I got pulled over somewhere in Ohio," I replied, somehow managing a smile.

"How fast were you going?"

"85."

Mom was so happy to have me home that she didn't even scold me, but I didn't care. I was just glad to not be in the car anymore. But then I grimaced as another sharp blow hit my belly, and I saw the worry on Mom's face.

"I'm exhausted," I said.

"Go ahead up," Mom said, nodding toward the stairs. "I made your bed. I'll be up in a few minutes."

I stood and took a deep breath before ascending the flight of stairs. They now looked as daunting as Longs Peak. I gripped the banister tightly as another stab took charge of my belly. Each step took more energy than the one before, and I felt like I would never reach the top.

"It's all in your head," I told myself as I closed my eyes, put one foot in front of the other and made it to the top and into my bedroom.

I pulled back the fresh sheets on the bed, kicked off my flip-flops, and slowly climbed in as the next jab of pain took over my body.

"I made up the couch-bed," Mom said from within the darkness of my bedroom. I was 22 years old and my Mom was going to sleep in my room.

"Thanks," I mumbled into the pillow. And before I could say another word, I was fast asleep.

That night, I was jerked awake by the same pain that had plagued my abdomen for over seven months. The room was spinning, and thick, sour bile was clogging the back of my throat. I stumbled through the dark into the bathroom, flipped on the light and fell to my knees, leaning over the porcelain bowl just in time to feel the warm, rotten liquid ejecting from my body. The pain was horrific.

"Molly, are you alright?" Mom knelt over me with one palm on my forehead and the other caressing my hair. I closed my eyes and leaned back on my heels.

"I'll be OK, Mom. This happens all the time." When she gasped, I realized the absurdity of what I had just said. I was definitely not OK. Standing up, I looked at myself in the mirror. Oh, my God! Who was that girl? Her face was gray, with dark brownish-blue circles under her eyes, and a bit of vomit on her right cheek. I ran the water, flinching at the cold as it hit my face, and glanced back at the stranger in the mirror before going back to bed.

"Molly? Can I do anything?" Mom's voice trembled this time, as it passed through my throbbing head. The porcelain was cold against my cheek and I closed my eyes, not wanting to move.

"I'm OK," I whispered in a barely audible croak. "I told you, this happens all the time."

Her hand brushed my cheek. This was the second time in one night that I had thrown up. Something was different.

"Do you want me to take you to the emergency room?" she pleaded.

I took in a breath and held it, waiting for the pain to ease again, but it wouldn't.

"No. I'll be OK in the morning."

I closed my eyes and held still, clenching my teeth and still waiting. I wanted to sleep. I wanted the pain to stop. I wanted to throw up some more. I wanted to give up and die, but instead the night went on.

I woke again four more times. The third time, there was nothing left to release but yellow and acidy bile. By the fourth time, there wasn't even any of that. I'd heard horror stories about dry heaves, but this was much worse than it had ever been described to me. There was so much pain.

"Please let me take you to the emergency room," she begged. But I only closed my eyes and slept until the next bout.

I looked at the clock. 5:17 a.m. I closed my eyes and looked again. 8:11 a.m. Oh, God, the pain was unbearable. If I laid on my back, it stretched me out too much, but if I laid on my stomach there was too much pressure. I couldn't sleep. I couldn't sit. I couldn't stand. Everything hurt. I just wanted to die. I'd been living with this fucking pain in my belly so long, and now, on February 12, 1999, I couldn't take it anymore. I was ready to give up.

"Mom," I whispered. "Help."

Before I could say another word, Mom was at my side. She and Dad helped me down the stairs and into the garage. Where were we going? Oh, God, it hurt. "Please make it stop," I begged.

Where was I? I opened my eyes and felt the pavement moving beneath the tires. I was in the passenger's seat of Mom's new car with the seat reclined all the way back, She was driving. I couldn't sit up. It hurt too much. Where were we going? Why was it taking so long? I was so dizzy.

"Molly? Molly! Are you OK?"

I didn't answer. I couldn't answer. The pain was too excruciating. I raised my head and looked around, but nothing made sense. We were making so many turns. I couldn't tell where we were. I didn't even know how long we'd been driving. Where the hell was she taking me? The car slowed down. Oh, God, please. Now the car was stopping. The passenger door opened. Oh, God, please don't make me move.

Mom pulled my legs toward her and lifted me out of the car. She held me up as we walked into what looked like a clinic and then she sat me in a stiff, wicker chair in the waiting room. Then she went to the reception desk. A little boy stared at me. Fuck you, kid! Leave me alone! Everyone just leave me alone! Oh, God, make it stop!

"Molly McMaster?" the nurse called. No. Please don't make me move again. Mom pulled me out of the chair and helped me down the hall and into the examination room. There was a woman. What was happening? X-rays? I had already had those in Colorado. Please don't make me move anymore. I heard their voices and saw their mouths moving, but I couldn't talk back. I just wanted the hurting to stop. Please!

They laid me on an X-ray table. The woman pulled my shirt up and looked at my belly. Why did I have such a huge belly? What was growing inside of me?

It was dark, and the X-ray machine made long, slow noises and seemed to take forever. There were voices in the room. I could hear Mom again.

"...total blockage...to the hospital...may need surgery..."

Who were they talking about? Who needed surgery? What was happening? I had a blockage? What could possibly be in there?

We were walking again, through the lobby and then outside into the chilly air. I closed my eyes and let Mom lead me. Where were we going next? Why hadn't they fixed me? The pain was still there, and it was getting worse.

"Molly?" Mom said loudly. "Can you hear me?"

"Uh huh," I nodded.

"We're going to the emergency room. You're going to be OK." She helped me into the car and slammed the door.

After the car came to a halt, I lifted my eyes and saw a young man in green scrubs, opening my door and helping me into a wheelchair. He wheeled me through the waiting room and through some heavy doors. The young man helped me onto an examining table. Mom and Dad were both there. Who was the other guy? He looked like the guy from that movie *Honey, I Shrunk the Kids*. What was his name? Rick Moranis? Oh, God, he wants me to talk to him.

"Molly, I'm Dr. Yarze. I'm a gastroenterologist. What's going on with you today?"

I couldn't answer. I tried, but I couldn't get the words out.

Mom spoke up. "We just came from the Moreau Health Clinic. They took some X-rays and told me to bring her here immediately."

A nurse came in and stabbed me with a needle, and within a few moments, the pain dulled to an almost tolerable state.

"Couldn't wait to see me, huh?" Aimee said, sticking her head into my examining room. I hadn't seen my brother's girlfriend since Christmas and was comforted just hearing her voice. She had recently added a few more letters to the end of her name, becoming a nurse practitioner, and had started a new job in another wing of Glens Falls Hospital only the week before.

Aimee sat with Mom and me for a few minutes before heading out to the nurse's station to get more information. When she returned, she explained that I would need to have an NG tube.

"What's that?" I asked from my semi-conscious state.

"I can tell you right now that you're not going to like it," she said. "It's uncomfortable but you need to have it, and the sooner you get it, the sooner your belly will feel better." The shot had somewhat numbed the pain, but my belly still seemed to be growing, and with it, the sharp stabbing. "The nurse will come in and insert it into your nose and push it all the way down into your stomach to suck out the bad stuff."

I began to cry. "Will it help?"

"Yes."

"Would you put it in for me?"

She was startled. "I could, but I don't think you'd ever speak to me again."

"Please, Aimee?" I begged. "I'd rather you put it in than anyone else."

"OK. If you promise you'll still talk to me when it's over."

I nodded and she left the room, reappearing a few minutes later with another nurse and a long, skinny hose. The nurse fretted around the room for a few minutes and then she asked everyone to leave except Aimee. I was feeling somewhat woozy as I watched Aimee fiddle with the tube.

"Are you ready?"

I nodded and she put a warm hand on my forehead and inserted the tube into my right nostril with the other. I began to gag while the hose scratched its way down the back of my throat. "I need you to swallow," she said as I choked on the tube. "Hang on." I was going to throw up. "Keep swallowing. We're almost done. There," she said. "We're in." My belly didn't feel any better.

Aimee stood up and connected the open end of a hose that was at least four feet long to a large clear bucket on the wall. It looked like an extra-large version of one of Mom's liquid measuring cups, with red lines and numbers on the side. There was another tube connected at one end to the clear bucket and at the other to a silver socket on the wall, which began a low hissing sound when it was turned on. Within a few moments, greenish goop and air bubbles began to rise up the tube from my stomach and were ejected via my right nostril. The stuff collected in the bucket attached to the wall. It was truly disgusting.

Aimee was right. The NG tube was one of the most uncomfortable experiences of my life, aside from the pain that I was already experiencing. But she was also right about the pressure in my belly easing as the tube suctioned green goop and air. I could still feel the tube rubbing against the back of my throat, and after a while it became uncomfortable to talk.

A few hours with the NG tube and my belly felt much better.

"When can we take it out?" I asked Aimee.

"Not yet," she said.

"When?" I asked again.

"Let's wait and talk to the doctor," she said. I had no idea that the tube would remain lodged in my throat for the next five days.

After a while, "Dr. Rick Moranis" came into the room and explained what was going to happen. I didn't listen, nor did I much care.

"As long as you can get me on a plane on Monday morning, Doc. I'm going to Florida to visit my big brother in Daytona Beach for my birthday, and I don't want to miss it."

Everyone just stared at me.

That afternoon, after various tests, a slightly receding belly and less pain than I'd felt in months, I was admitted to the hospital. I needed emergency surgery, so Mom, Dad and I chose Dr. Thompson, a neighbor and family friend who had operated on Dad more than once. The procedure was scheduled for early the next morning, and finally it began to sink in. There would be no Florida, and I wasn't going anywhere. Something was seriously wrong.

The next day I was startled as I awoke and felt my bed moving beneath me. Where was I? I was rolled down a long corridor and had no idea where I was going. My bed stopped next to a wall. I stared up at the ceiling light and wondered if this was what prison was like: silence and boredom. A man wearing a stethoscope and pale green scrubs approached me.

"Good morning, Molly."

He was adorable. But how did he know my name? Maybe he had asked someone. Maybe he wanted my phone number.

"How are you feeling this morning?"

"OK," I croaked, trying to clear my dry throat, but then remembering the NG tube.

"I'm your anesthesiologist," he continued. "We're prepping you for surgery."

I wanted to sink into my pillow as I realized that I hadn't showered since Grandma's house two or three days earlier. Besides, the handsome doctor didn't want my phone number. He just wanted me to sleep!

I woke after surgery and saw Mom and Dad in my room talking with Dr. Thompson, but everything was blurry, and I was tired. I closed my eyes and began to dream.

PART II

CANCER

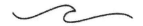

"More than anything else, I believe it's our decisions, not the conditions of our lives, that determine our destiny."

Anthony Robbins

8

DIAGNOSIS

▲

When I finally woke from my haze, the salty aroma of soup hung in the air, and a nurse held my wrist, taking my pulse. I really was in the hospital.

An IV pole was dripping a bag of clear fluid into my right arm. But I did a double-take when I saw the other contraption tethered to my left arm. This one looked like something out of *Star Wars*. A large, electric blue box with blinking numbers and lights fastened to a slim metal pole – a skinny, baby-blue R2-D2. My eyes followed a thick, gray cord to a plug in the wall, and I realized I couldn't move too far from the bed. My eyes shifted back to R2-D2 and the two upside-down bottles that oozed different liquids – one milky white, the other clear and yellowish. Later I would find out that one bottle was filled with lipids, a fancy way to say fats, and the other with electrolytes. I was so malnourished that I needed to be fed intravenously, but this wasn't like a normal IV. The one in my left arm was called a PICC line (peripherally inserted central catheter), and actually ran through a vein and up my arm to my heart. I needed nourishment right at the source, I guess.

"Those bottles probably contain the most expensive meal you'll ever have," Dad joked. "Make sure you enjoy them."

Looking down at my belly, and even from under a blanket, it seemed flatter than it had been the day before. The pain was still there, but it was different now. The severe pressure was gone, and in its place was a raw, stinging sensation that turned into a raging burn when I tried to roll onto my side. Lying flat on my back, I pulled the covers to one side and was relieved by what I saw. An oversized Ace bandage was wrapped around my entire waist, covering whatever had happened there that morning.

"How are you feeling?" the nurse asked. I nodded, still a little bit woozy. "I'll be back in a little bit to check on you." She took my blood pressure, opened the privacy curtain to reveal Mom and Dad, then left the room.

"How are you doing?" Mom asked, moving toward me.

"OK," I croaked, surprised to feel the NG tube still clogging the back of my throat. "I'm a little bit lightheaded." I reached up and touched my nose. "And when can this thing come out?"

"I'll ask Aimee." Mom sat down on the edge of my bed and ran her fingers through my hair.

"Where is everyone? Who was here earlier?"

"Dad and I have been here all morning, and Aimee came a few hours ago," she said. "Kristina ran into some of your friends from high school. They wanted to see you."

I managed a small smile, remembering Brian and A.C.'s voices. So that hadn't been a dream.

"Dr. Thompson wants you to get as much rest as you can today," Dad said. "He wants you out of bed as early as tomorrow. Probably have you running a marathon with him by the end of the week."

Dr. Thompson didn't have me running any marathons, but soon I was hanging onto both IV poles and walking the hallways as much as possible in my revealing backless gown. When I wasn't meandering the halls, I had strict orders to blow into a blue Slinky-like tube attached to another clear vertical tube with a ball at the bottom. When I blew into it, the ball would rise.

"It's so you don't get pneumonia," Dr. Thompson said sternly one morning.

"But it *hurts*," I whined.

"I know it *hurts*," he said, playfully mimicked my bratty voice, "but if you get pneumonia, you're going to be here a lot longer."

"Yes, sir." When I blew into the tube hard enough to make the ball rise at the other end, I felt like my abdominal muscles would pop right out, but Dr. Thompson stood over me, making sure I did it correctly.

"When can I get something to eat?" I finally asked.

"Not until the NG tube comes out."

"Well, when can *that* come out?"

"When we know your bowels are working properly again."

"What? Are they on strike or something?"

"Sort of," he laughed. "You just had major surgery. We had to reattach your intestine, and because of that, your bowels have basically been paralyzed for a little while. It's called ileus."

"That's gross," I said.

"That's why I'm in here so often listening to your belly with my stethoscope. I'm listening for the noises the intestines make when they're working again."

I thought back to the day when my belly made those loud "cat noises" during my college class.

"When you pass gas for the first time, tell the nurse and they'll disconnect your NG tube from suction for a while. If you don't get sick, we'll take it out completely."

"All I have to do is *fart*?" I asked.

"Yes."

"And then I can eat?"

"We'll start you on a liquid diet. Soup, Jell-O, juice."

"And how long does it usually take?"

"It will be a few more days," he said with a smile.

I rolled my eyes and let out a frustrated sigh. How I longed to chew on a slice of greasy New York style pizza!

"You've got a lot of friends thinking of you, Moll," he said, changing the subject and inclining his head at the flowers lined up on the windowsill and placed on nearly every available flat surface.

As the days wore on, I walked a little farther and floated the ball a little longer. Although I had 32 metal staples in my skin that kept the 10-inch vertical incision from bursting open, the pain was finally lessening. Now the stabbing pain that I endured for months was almost gone. It almost didn't feel real.

"Hey, Moe. Did you fart yet?" Seeking maximum embarrassment, Kristina asked that question each time she visited me.

"Not yet," I replied each time. But then the moment I anxiously awaited finally came.

"Can we take it out now?" I begged the nurse. Because my intestines were working again, my NG tube had been unhooked from the suction on the wall and clamped off, just as Dr. Thompson had promised.

"You can leave it in there if she's driving you nuts," Dad said.

"How long has it been unhooked?" she asked.

"Eight hours," I lied. I had been watching the minute hand on the clock since the moment they had unhooked me from the wall, and knew I had 14 more minutes to go. "Please?"

"Are you feeling sick or anything?" she asked.

"No. I feel great, except for this stupid tube in my throat!"

"Alright," the nurse said. She pulled a pair of rubber gloves from a box on the wall.

"Will it hurt?" I asked.

"Well, there are probably other things you'd rather do with your time," she said.

The nurse peeled the white medical tape off my nose. It had held the NG tube in place for five days.

"Are you ready?" the nurse asked.

"Yeah."

"I need you to take a nice deep breath. When I count to three, you're going to exhale it all back out, nice and hard, OK?"

"One. Two. Three," she counted, and I began to blow out hard through my nose and mouth. I gagged as I felt something slicing higher and higher up the back of my throat. When I felt the scratchy end that had been lodged in my stomach reach the top of my throat, I knew it was almost over. But at the very last moment, I felt a pop and excruciating pain. I sobbed and grabbed my nose just as the nurse cleared the end of the tube from my nostril.

She didn't say anything, just walked away with the tube in her hand. I was certain that my nasal passage had ruptured. I rocked back and forth in my bed, crying, then took my hands from my face to check for blood, but there was none. As the pain subsided, I realized that Dad was sitting on the edge of the bed, holding me, rocking with me.

I was 10 years old when Mom and Dad brought Rob and me along to Ohio for Dad's high school reunion. We stayed with Grandma and Grandpa in the old house on the river. I don't remember Grandpa's heart attack that week, but I vividly remember running up the long gravel driveway one sunny afternoon to flag down the ambulance. As I looked at Dad, holding and rocking me, I realized that this was only the second time I'd ever seen him cry.

The next day, there was a very special delivery.

"Hi, Judy!" I said excitedly. I hadn't seen Jason's mother for years. Jason was my brother's best friend and was like a second brother to me, which meant twice the teasing. But today, from behind her back, Judy pulled out a brand-new hockey stick tied with ribbons and balloons. "Jason thought you might like it!" She smiled and handed the stick to me.

"Thank you so much!" I said, beaming and realizing that this was the first time I had thought about hockey since the night I left Colorado. Jason's gift was my first reminder of what I was supposed to be doing.

"I can't wait to try it out!" I said.

That afternoon, I talked one of the nurses into unplugging R2-D2 and giving me a roll of medical tape, which I unwound, balled up and batted around in the hallway like a puck. I looked ridiculous in my backless nightie, moving timidly around so as not to disturb the staples in my belly and wheeling two IV poles, but Dr. Thompson was happy that I was out of bed and I could finally feel my passion coming back.

On February 19, 1999, my 23rd birthday and six days after surgery, Dr. Thompson told me about my cancer. He said they had removed twenty-five inches of my large intestine and held up his fists to show me the size.

"I've never seen anyone so young with colon cancer," he said. "You're probably the only one in the country to be diagnosed this young - maybe even the world." The possibility that I had cancer had never even crossed my mind.

Dr. Thompson dropped the bomb and left. Then Mom and Dad entered. It was obvious that they had both been crying and were badly shaken. Why did they already know? I didn't want them to know. I didn't want anyone to know. I felt sick and weak. People would never again treat me as the confident, hockey-playing Molly that it had taken me 23 years to find. Instead, I would forever be known as "Molly with cancer." As the thoughts dribbled through my mind, I couldn't hold back tears. How could I have cancer?

Mom sat on the edge of my bed and tried to take my hand, but I pulled away. I wanted her to leave. I wanted them both to leave.

"Why do you already know?" I snapped angrily, tears streaking my cheeks. "Who told you?"

"We spoke with Dr. Thompson in the hallway," Dad replied softly.

"He should have told me first! It's none of your business!" I was enraged. How could he have told anyone else before me? I was the patient. It was my decision who knew.

"Molly, he's a friend of the family," Mom said. "He really didn't know what to do."

"He told us that he got it all," Dad said.

"He also said it was unheard of in someone your age," Mom said.

"I don't care," I snapped. "He still should have told me first. Now you're going to tell everyone."

"You don't want anyone to know?" Mom quickly asked.

"No!"

"Molly, you're going to be OK," Dad said.

"Do you want us to leave you alone?" Mom asked, cutting him off.

"Yes!" I sobbed. "Just go away!"

Dad took Mom's hand and they reluctantly left me alone. I cried and questions raced through my head. How could this have happened? How could I have cancer?

Then the phone rang. I covered my ears. It rang again and again. I didn't want to answer it because I didn't want to tell anyone that I was sick and could die. Finally, I picked up the receiver.

"Happy birthday, Moll!"

"Hi, Rock," I whispered. I smiled for a brief second. He always seemed to know when I needed a laugh.

"How ya' feelin?"

"OK, I guess. What are you doing?" I wanted to talk about anything but cancer. I wanted to abandon my world and live in his.

"Talkin' to you, Clown! 'Whatsa matta'?" The soreness in the back of my throat returned as I fought against tears. I couldn't tell him. But maybe if I did, Rocky would treat me like a normal person.

"Nothing." My voice was getting higher.

"Are you crying? There's no crying in baseball!" he commanded. I managed a slight giggle. "C'mon, Moll. Seriously, 'whatsa matta'?"

I took a deep breath. "It's serious, Rock. The surgery I had."

"No kiddin'. They opened up 'ya' stomach."

I smiled again, knowing that he was trying to make me laugh."

"Rock," I said, the tears falling. "I have cancer."

"*What?*" I couldn't tell if he was shocked or really hadn't heard me.

"I have colon cancer." I had trouble saying the words. I was talking about cancer and my colon in the same sentence. He probably thought I was disgusting.

"What does that mean?"

"I…I'm not really sure," I was openly crying, but it felt good to tell someone. It felt good to tell him. "My doctor said I'm going to be OK, but who knows?" I was sharing the weight of my horrible disease. "I'll probably have to do chemotherapy." Until that moment, the chemo hadn't even hit me. I was pretty sure that Dr. Thompson had mentioned it. But when the words left my lips, I began to see my future, and I didn't see any hockey. I was terrified.

"Wow," Rocky said. "That *sucks*."

"Thanks," I said, managing a smile. I appreciated his bluntness.

"Molly, I really don't know what to say to you." I'd never heard him speak so seriously. "I've never been through anything like this, so I can't tell you how or what you should be feeling. I won't pretend that I can, but I do know one thing."

"What's that?" I asked.

"You're going to make it through this. You'll beat it because you're strong – you're Molly."

I floated through the rest of the day in a haze of confusion and sadness, not mentioning my cancer to anyone who entered the room. But when a raspberry Jell-O birthday cake arrived, I knew I had to call my brother. Rob had worked at this hospital for a few years and knew who to call for a favor. Now he was following his dream to become a commercial airline pilot. I wanted to play ice hockey in the Olympics, but I had cancer instead. I couldn't even look at the cake. But I called my brother anyway, hoping he wouldn't notice that I'd been crying.

When I was in high school, Rob was on the rowing team at Ithaca College. A few days before my 16th birthday, when he was home for a visit, he invited me to go to the gym with him. I had nearly fallen over! I had always looked up to my brother and would have done anything to spend time with him. Instead, I was the annoying little sister. When Rob invited me to go with him that night, I didn't care that it was 10:30 at night. I didn't care that I still had homework, or that I had school in the morning. With a huge smile, I jumped into his little yellow sports car.

At the gym, Rob showed me how the ergometer worked as he rowed, and he explained what a coxswain was. He told me about his team and his races and tried to sell me on rowing. After 45 minutes, we headed toward the parking lot.

"Wanna drive?" he asked.

"Yeah, right."

"Seriously." He held up the keys.

"Rob, I'm not 16 yet," I said. "I don't even have a permit."

"Close enough. Isn't your birthday in a few days?"

"It's one thing to drive the Jeep up and down the dirt road at the lake but kind of another to drive in town."

"Whatever," he said, tossing the keys across the parking lot. I froze. Was he serious? Or was this like the time he piled Hershey's Kisses on the table and asked me if I wanted a chocolate kiss. Of course I did, so he put a Hershey's Kiss in his mouth, chewed it up a bit and then kissed me on the cheek.

"Rob, C'mon," I said.

"Molly, it's no big deal." He was standing at the passenger door of his car. "Unlock the door, will ya? It's cold."

I unlocked the doors and slid into the driver's seat. "Are you sure?" I asked, giving him one last out.

"Just drive. Let's go the long way."

Rob directed me across town and then onto I-87, the expressway that travels north to Canada. When I pulled to a stop in the driveway at home, I turned and looked at my big brother.

"Not bad," he said.

I smiled from ear to ear. "Thank you," I said.

He wasn't teasing me the way he usually did, and I wasn't pestering him. Instead, we sat together and shared one of the first grownup memories I have with my brother. On that day, we were equals.

"What's going on up there?"

Rob's voice on the phone pulled me back to my stark hospital room.

"Nothing." I wanted to tell him but didn't know how. He wasn't as easy to talk to as Rocky was, and there hadn't been many of those grown up moments since the night I drove his car.

"Nothing? Aimee says your room is filled with flowers, and you've had so many visitors that the nurses had to finally start kicking people out." Aimee and her two boys had flown down to visit Rob the day before. It was the trip we were all supposed to be on, but thanks to my stupid cancer, Mom, Dad and I were spending my birthday in the hospital instead. I had to tell him about my cancer, but I couldn't get the words out.

"Did you get your cake?" he asked.

"Um, yeah. Thank you." The words just wouldn't budge from my lips. Why couldn't I tell him?

"Um, Rob, I ..." It was on the edge of my tongue. I was ready.

"Yeah?" he asked.

"Um, I..." I hesitated again. I chickened out. I just couldn't say the words "I have cancer."

"OK," he said. "Happy birthday and get better soon."

"Thanks, Rob. I love you."

"Love you too."

"Hello? How are ya?'" Aimee's voice was on the line.

"Better," I lied. "My NG tube finally came out. I farted and it was like a big party in here."

"Congratulations. That means your insides are working again."

"Yeah, and now everyone on the floor knows that I farted." I managed a slight giggle. Aimee laughed. If I told her, she could tell Rob.

"Molly, are you OK? Is there something you want to tell me?"

"No. I mean yes. I have colon cancer," I finally whispered.

"Oh, shit," Aimee said, startled.

"I couldn't tell Rob." I was sobbing again. "I wanted to, but I just couldn't, and I don't know why."

"It's OK. Do you want to talk to him again?"

"No. I can't."

"Do you want me to tell him?" she asked.

"I think so."

"I can do that," she said. "Molly, you're going to be OK. I've been reading my medical books ever since I found out about the tumor, and the more I read, the more I felt like I was sinking on the Titanic."

"Why didn't you tell me?" I whispered.

"Molly, I wanted to. I wanted to scream out but couldn't. You weren't my patient. And what if I had been wrong?"

I was silent.

"Did they test any lymph nodes?" she finally asked.

"I heard Dr. Thompson saying something about 11 of them. They were all negative. What does that mean?"

"Molly, that's great news! That means your cancer was probably caught before it spread."

"Thanks, Aimee." I knew she wanted me to believe that, but I thought I heard uncertainty in her voice.

Just then, a new face appeared in my room.

"Hi, Molly. I'm Sam from the Oncology department, and I just wanted to come up and tell you how strong and brave I think you are." *Strong? Brave?* Aren't those things you choose to be? I didn't choose cancer, and I sure as hell wasn't brave!

That evening, when Mom and Dad went home to get some sleep, Kristina arrived with her Monopoly board.

"Doubles! Ha! Ha! I get to go again," she said, snatching the dice from the board. The bed next to mine creaked as my roommate got up and left the room. I knew that if I was going to tell Kristina the bad news, now would be the best time. I'd been waiting all day for this moment and had changed my mind dozens of times. Should I tell her? I couldn't shake that "poor Molly with cancer" feeling, but after talking with Rocky and Aimee, I decided I wanted my best friend to know.

I looked at Kristina. "Um, Tee." My eyes were beginning to water, and the room was getting warmer.

"Yeah?" She looked up at me and put the dice down, realizing that I was about to reveal something important.

"I'm going to tell you something serious." I took a long, slow breath. "But I don't want you to ever repeat it, and I don't ever want to talk about it again – *ever*. OK?"

"Umm, OK." She looked frightened.

I tried to stall but couldn't find anything else to say. Why was it so difficult? Finally, I counted to three and blurted it out. "I have colon cancer." Tears poured down my cheeks. Kristina sobbed too. I wanted to hug her and tell her what Aimee had said, that I was going to be OK, but, at that exact moment, I heard the skittering of slippers. My roommate reappeared in the doorway, and I wiped the tears from my eyes. Looking directly into my eyes, Kristina picked up the dice and rolled them without another word.

As I slowly got my strength back, the nurses allowed more visitors, and it seemed like the more people I told about my cancer, the better I felt, as if I was sharing the burden of my disease. Some people were treating me the way I was afraid they would, as "poor helpless Molly," but most treated me the same as they always had.

Mom and Kristina took turns spending the night with me, and each day my walks got longer and longer. At first, I walked to the end of the hall, but only when I was supervised. Then I started walking all the way around the corridor and sometimes around the entire floor. Sometimes I took my new hockey stick and sometimes I didn't. One day I was caught taking the elevator to the lobby.

Finally, the day came. Nine days after my surgery, with a reluctant but sincere promise to Dr. Thompson that I wouldn't drive myself *anywhere* for at least four weeks, the nurse wheeled me out of my room.

"I can walk, you know." I told her confidently.

"I know, but the hospital rules state that a patient being discharged has to go in a wheelchair."

"Hold on!" Kristina said. She grabbed my wrist and tied a balloon on to my arm. "There," she giggled. "Much better."

I glanced up at the red, metallic balloon over my head. "Hooray! I farted!" was handwritten in fat, dark letters.

"Thanks," I said, trying desperately to untie Kristina's quadruple knot. I held my hand over my face all the way down the elevator and halfway across the lobby. But did it really matter? Pooping. Farting. Both were things that people did every day. During my hospital stay, everyone who entered the room seemed to be interested in how my bowels were operating. With the balloon still tied tightly around my wrist, I realized that *not* talking about my bowels over the past few months had nearly killed me. I let the hand that concealed my face fall into my lap, and I owned that red balloon.

9

DR. MARTELO

On February 23, three days after I left the hospital, Mom, Dad and I returned to meet with Dr. Martelo, my new oncologist. I simply called him "my cancer doc."

"Good morning, Molly," he said in a soft accent that I couldn't quite place. He closed the door behind him and smiled warmly.

"How are you feeling?"

"OK," I said.

"Are you having any trouble with the incision?" He nodded at my belly.

"No. Seems OK."

"Good." He nodded again, sat down on a rolling stool and dropped a thick file folder on the table in front of me. My eyes widened as I took note of the fat medical history I had racked up in just two weeks.

"What we've got here," he began, flipping through the pages in the file and looking at Mom and Dad, "is Dukes B, Stage two adenocarcinoma."

Who the heck was Duke?

"You were very lucky." He looked at me and then back at my parents. "The cancer made it through the entire bowel wall and to the outside where it was touching other organs, but all 11 lymph nodes that we tested came back negative."

"Aimee told me that was good," I blurted.

"It is good," Dr. Martelo said. "It means that your cancer was contained. It hasn't spread, which is when it really becomes a problem. Another few weeks, and your story may not have turned out the same."

"What do you mean?" I asked.

"Another few weeks, and the cancer might have found its way into those lymph nodes. Once that happens, the likelihood of recurrence goes up and survival rates drop significantly." He turned to face my parents once again. I found myself growing more and more irritated each time he turned away from me, the patient, to speak to them.

"What about treatment?" Dad asked.

"That's a choice you can make. Because the cancer was contained, chemotherapy may not be necessary. However, because of Molly's age, I would recommend that she receive treatment anyway."

"Why?" Dad asked.

I wanted Dad to be quiet so that I could ask the questions. There I was, 23 years old and still feeling like a child.

"Mr. McMaster, the form of colon cancer that Molly had was very slow growing. If she were 80 years old, I would not recommend chemotherapy since we're quite sure the total of it was removed during surgery. If it ever came back, she would likely have already died of old age. However, because of her youth, even though it was caught early enough and the likelihood of it coming back is very low, I don't think we should take any chances."

I was getting more and more annoyed as he directed his answers toward Mom and Dad.

"What is the chemotherapy like?" Mom asked.

"That's where we're lucky. There are over 50 different chemotherapy drugs today, and the one we would recommend for Molly is extremely tolerable."

"Fifty different colon cancer drugs?" Mom asked. I silently wished they would leave the room.

"No. Fifty different chemotherapy drugs. There are many different types of cancer. Colon. Breast. Lung. Cervical. Those are just a few. Each one of them requires a different treatment, and some of those treatments are much harsher than the one we will recommend for Molly."

"Will I lose my hair?" I piped up, trying to get his attention.

Dr. Martelo turned to face me. "There's always the chance that you'll lose your hair, but most patients don't react that way to this form of treatment."

"And what drugs are you recommending?" Dad was scribbling madly on a pad he brought from home.

"I'm going to prescribe two drugs. One is called 5-FU, which is the actual chemotherapy, and the other is called leucovorin, which is a vitamin B derivative that will enhance the effects of the chemotherapy. That's the standard treatment for Molly's stage of cancer."

"And how long will that last?" Dad asked.

"I would normally have you do six, six-week cycles, but a recent study has shown that four six-week cycles works just as well."

"So, does that mean six or four?" I asked.

"Probably four cycles of six weeks each, so 24 weeks, but I'd like you to see a doctor at Dana-Farber Cancer Institute in Boston for a second opinion."

"And what's this chemo going to be like?" I quickly asked before anyone else could speak again.

"Molly, the form of chemotherapy that you will get, if you opt for treatment, has minimal side effects. Your sense of taste will probably change, and your energy level will go down. You may experience nausea and maybe some vomiting. You'll probably have some diarrhea, but those are all very mild."

"But I probably won't lose my hair?" I asked again.

"Probably not," he said. "Basically, if you do opt for treatment, I want you to go about the next year of your life like you would any other year." He smiled sweetly at me as though he'd just given me a wonderful gift. Instead, my heart surged in my chest and my face got hot, but I couldn't tell if it was out of rage or sadness.

"Molly, are you OK?" he asked. "Molly?" he repeated softly.

"No, I'm not OK!" I shouted through boiling tears. "I don't have *years* like everyone else! The next *year* of my life was supposed to be spent training for a hockey tryout in Canada!" I was angry, hurt and unable to control myself.

The room was silent. Mom and Dad glared at me, likely horrified at my behavior. Dr. Martelo finally broke the silence.

"Molly?" His voice was soft and soothing. "Are you mad at me?"

I shook my head slowly and then lowered it, ashamed of lashing out at him. It wasn't his fault that I'd gotten cancer. He smiled warmly and I couldn't help but smile back. I knew I would like him.

Mom, Dad and I decided to seek the recommended second opinion at Dana-Farber. We went home to wait for a call with an appointment date. Little did I know that chemo would have to wait. Once again, my belly had other plans.

Ten days after my surgery, Dr. Thompson walked his dog down to my parents' house and took my 32 staples out while I lay on the green couch in the living room. My healing was inching along.

"You'd better be walking," he said. "The more you move, the sooner you heal."

I had been moving some, but was more anxious to get out of the house than to exercise, so a few days after my staples came out, I joined Mom at Sunday morning church. I was not an avid churchgoer and my abdomen was still quite raw, but it seemed like a low-intensity option.

On the way to church, as Mom and I chatted in the car, I felt pain in my belly somewhat like I had experienced in Colorado, but not nearly as severe. I ignored it, assuming it was just part of my recovery, but less than an hour later and only halfway through the sermon, the stabbing became so sharp that I couldn't sit any longer. I stood up in the pew and walked down the aisle as fast as someone who had just had major abdominal surgery could go. I'll never know if it was from the pain or sheer panic that it was starting all over again, but halfway down the aisle I began to sob uncontrollably. I covered my mouth with one hand to silence myself and hid in the bathroom. Mom found me a few minutes later and we quickly drove home to call Dr. Thompson.

"Dr. Thompson says that the pain you are having is most likely adhesions," Mom said, as I lay sprawled on the couch. "He says it's normal and you should take it easy but keep walking."

"What's an adhesion?" I asked.

"It's when things stick together. He said it happens after surgery sometimes."

"Great," I said sarcastically. "So this is my new normal?" Did I give up one pain just to find another?

"He's leaving on a ski trip early in the morning but said that if you are still having trouble this week we should get in touch with his on-call doctor."

"I'm OK," I said, standing up from the couch and feeling slightly better. "I'm sure it's just my insides starting to work again," I said, more for my own benefit.

But the next day, I knew that wasn't the case.

Kristina and I sat across from each other in the living room playing another game of Monopoly.

"Get your dirty paws off my dice," I said, snatching them from the board. I held a pillow over my belly, finding the light pressure comforting. The pillow helped me *not* feel like my insides might fall out at any moment.

"Ouch!" I cried out, grabbing at and pushing down on the lower part of my abdomen.

"Are you OK?" Kristina asked, startled into seriousness.

I gritted my teeth and sucked in air, hoping to relieve the pain, but it didn't help. Tears were brimming in my eyes. "Can you get my Mom?" I gasped.

Kristina and Mom helped me to the car, and we hurried back to the emergency room.

"They put you in the Can't Decide Unit, huh Mokins?" Dad asked later that afternoon. He didn't think much of the CDU, also known as the Critical Decision Unit, where I had been admitted for observation.

I tried to laugh, but throughout the day the pain had only gotten worse. Dr. Thompson's backup doctor had been in half a dozen times but couldn't pinpoint the problem. He stuck with Dr. Thompson's original adhesions idea and sent me for X-rays. I was prescribed morphine, but that didn't touch the pain. As day turned into night, it became more and more excruciating. I couldn't escape it. All night long I pushed the button for morphine, and all night long the stabbing continued over and over and over again. I was ready to give up. Then around three a.m., the nurse asked for a higher dose of morphine, and I got a little bit of unbroken sleep.

"I figured it out!" Dr. Burns nearly shouted as he burst through the door. I squinted through puffy and bloodshot eyes at the clock. It was just past 6:30 in the morning. "I was in the shower this morning and realized what's going on," he said too excitedly. "Your *bowel* has died!"

I hated him. I hated his voice. I hated his excitement over dead bowel, and more than anything I hated his bedside manner. He was cocky and rude and not like Dr. Thompson at all.

"Please make it stop hurting," I begged him through gritted teeth and more tears.

"You'll need to go in for another surgery this morning," he said.

"Noooo. Please, No," I cried. "I can't go through it again."

"Molly, we need to open you up again and cut the dead part out," he said matter-of-factly.

"*Please*," I begged. "I don't want another NG tube." Now Mom's eyes began to water.

"Molly, the longer it's like that, the more toxic it will get. We need to take it out."

"Please, no!" I begged again. "Please no NG tube," I repeated through sobs.

"The nurses will prep you for surgery shortly," he said, and then he was gone. Mom put her arms around me and together we cried.

In less than an hour, my bed rolled along the corridor toward the operating room for the second time in just two and a half weeks. I wasn't even fully recovered, yet I was about to go through it all again.

When I woke from the anesthesia, I felt the familiar burn in my belly again, and I lifted my hand to my nose to find another NG tube. Panic rose from my toes and I found myself only able to take short labored breaths. If I began to cry, the pain would be unbearable so soon after surgery. Instead, I slowed my breathing. In through the nose. Out through the mouth. Each time the air filled my lungs, my heartbeat seemed to slow, until I felt calm.

It turned out that cocky Dr. Burns had been incorrect with his diagnosis. I did need that second surgery, but when he opened me back up, he found that my intestine had herniated itself. I also had adhesions and an abscess. He fixed the herniated intestine, cleaned me out thoroughly and started IV antibiotics. He also put some sort of medical silk between my organs so that they wouldn't adhere to themselves again. I spent another nine days in the hospital doing exactly what I had done a few weeks earlier, and prayed that I would never have to go through it again.

The recovery process was a little easier the second time around, and although Dr. Burns had told me I needed to wait at least six weeks before resuming even light activities, I felt strong at four weeks. I couldn't wait any longer, and a light skate couldn't possibly hurt. In the back of my car, I found my hockey skates in the pile of belongings that had traveled with me from Colorado, and against doctor's orders, drove myself to the local ice rink.

Sitting on a bench, my incision burned when I bent over to tie my skates. I stood and walked toward the ice, then skated around the rink a few times ever so slowly. I hadn't been on the ice in over two months, and I felt it. My balance was off, and my center of gravity was out of whack, possibly from the weight I had lost, but also from the awkward stance I had to keep to protect my irritated abdomen. Push. Glide. Push. Glide. The icy air felt wonderful in my lungs, and the breeze through my hair made me feel like I was back home. Push. Glide. Push. Glide. I don't know what it was about the sensation of skating, but it just felt right. I was meant to be on the ice.

Suddenly, I caught an edge of my skate blade in a groove in the ice and lost my balance. While it normally would have been easy to keep myself from falling, I couldn't stop and protect my still raw incision at once. I fell hard to my knees. Immediately, the incision felt like it was on fire and that my belly was ripping open.

I waited a few moments, breathing deeply to absorb the pains in my belly and knee, then stood up to see stars circling my head. I lifted my shirt and saw blood trickling from the incision. I left the rink and didn't go back to skate again until after my six-week window was up.

On St. Patrick's Day, I drove to Boston with Mom and Dad for an appointment at Dana-Farber Cancer

Institute, a principal teaching affiliate of Harvard's Medical School. I was relieved that the doctor recommended the same course of treatment that Dr. Martelo had prescribed. We left Dana-Farber more confident that I would survive my battle with colon cancer and celebrated with an early dinner, where I ordered my first-ever lobster, drenched in melted butter.

"You can do your treatments here in Boston or at the cancer center in Glens Falls with Dr. Martelo," Dad said. "Do you want to do them here?"

I thought about Dr. Martelo and the nurses that I had met so far. They were so kind, and I was very comfortable with them, despite my initial irritation with Dr. Martelo when he directed his gaze and comments at my parents and not me, the patient.

Then there was the driving. Being in a car four hours each way once a week for the next six months wasn't appealing. Would I do it alone? Would someone come with me each week? What if I was sick from chemo? I cracked a smile as I realized the absurdity of my thoughts. The drive was the inconvenience, not the cancer.

I thought about my parents. It drove me crazy when Dr. Martelo spoke to them and not to me, as though I was a child who couldn't handle her cancer. In Boston, Dr. Fuchs turned and looked directly at me when answering questions, no matter who was asking them.

I looked across the table. I loved my parents so much, and as strong as I wanted to pretend I was, I knew I could never do this without them. Who was I kidding? I needed them and doing my treatment in Glens Falls was the logical way to be sure that they were there.

"I want to stay at home," I said, taking the last bite of my delicious lobster, "and I want to start next week. The sooner I start, the sooner I'll be able to put cancer behind me forever."

10

TREATMENT

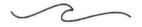

A few days before my first chemotherapy treatment, Sarah came to visit and brought me a small box tied with a red bow.

"What's this?" I asked, untying the bow and tearing the paper.

"Just a little something that I want you to have," she said.

Inside the box was a pewter charm engraved with a Chinese symbol, hanging from a black cord.

"Courage," Sarah said, answering the question I was preparing to ask.

"I love it. Thank you, Sar." I tied it around my neck and gave her a hug. Just like the tape she made for me before I left for Colorado, the necklace would become a source of strength when I couldn't find it on my own.

My first chemotherapy treatment was almost fun. I had a 9:00 a.m. appointment at the Glens Falls Hospital, so at 8:30 a.m., I laced up my in-line skates and rolled out of the house wearing my new necklace.

"I'll meet you there!" Mom yelled as I rolled down the driveway. It was only a 15-minute skate, and the crisp spring air felt wonderful on my face. Over two months, I'd been diagnosed with cancer and had two surgeries, yet there I was cruising around in the sunshine. It was good to be alive.

I rolled into the brightly lit lobby of the hospital's Charles R. Wood Cancer Center and saw Mom waiting with a bagel and juice.

After a few minutes, it was time for a blood draw, and I skated into a small white room near the front desk that smelled of rubbing alcohol. The lab technician gave me a funny look but didn't ask about my wheels. Instead, she stuck me with the first of what would become dozens and dozens of needles.

"What do you test my blood for?" I asked innocently.

"We do a CEA and a CBC," she said.

"Oh, and what are those?"

"Sorry," she laughed. "CEA stands for carcinoembryonic antigen, and it's a tumor marker test. If it goes up, it's a sign that the cancer may be back. And CBC is a complete blood count. It tests your white and red blood cells."

"And what do those tests mean?"

"If your red count goes down, it means you're anemic. If your white goes up, it means you have an infection, and if it goes down, it means that your immune system isn't up to par, so you may not be able to receive your chemotherapy."

"Why not?"

"If you get an infection, your body won't be able to fight it off."

"What happens if I can't get treatment?" I asked.

"Normally you just take a week off, and when you come in the following week we test again. The counts usually go back up by then."

"And it's OK to skip a week?"

"Sure," she said as she stuck a Band-Aid to my arm.

Rolling back into the lobby to await the test results, I vowed that no matter what happened, I would never allow my white count to go down. I wanted to get this over with as soon as possible, and low counts would only drag it out.

After 15 minutes and people casting strange looks at my skates, a nurse came into the lobby and called my name. Mom walked next to me as I rolled into the "chemo lobby," where most patients sat together and received their treatment. I chose one of the pink reclining chairs that lined the wall, sat down and propped my feet up with my skates still on.

"I'm here!" I announced. "Stick me!"

"Cut that out," Mom scolded.

"Hold on. We've got to find a good vein first," the nurse said, tapping two fingers along the inside of my arm. "OK, here's one." I looked away and grimaced. "Here we go," she said, and I felt a sharp stab as the needle went in.

"Ouch!"

"Did that hurt?" she asked.

"A little bit," I admitted.

"Oh, come on. It wasn't that bad. Are you afraid of blood too?" she asked.

"Only my own."

She pulled something away and attached a short, clear rubber tube to where the needle had gone into my arm. Then she taped everything to my skin, leaving only a small amount of tube visible, and a round, blue stub about the size of the end of my pinky finger. "I'll be right back with your treatment."

I glanced around the room at the other patients. Most of them sat quietly alone, and each was attached to the same electric blue *Star Wars* IV pole that I was introduced to during my first hospital stay. Some of them were sleeping with their feet propped up in their pink recliners. Two of them were sipping juice from small cans, the kind that a flight attendant might hand out. Some had hair and some didn't. Of the ones who didn't, most wore bandannas or hats. Some looked frail, others did not. And then, all at once, it hit me. No one in the room appeared to be under the age of 60, and except for me, no one was smiling.

"Are you going to eat your bagel?" Mom asked.

I felt guilty as I looked at the patients around me. They were probably nauseated and couldn't eat anything.

"I'm going to wait a little bit," I said, even though my stomach was churning, and some food might have settled it.

When the nurse returned, she was wheeling my own *Star Wars* IV pole, and hanging from the top was a bag filled with clear liquid.

"This is the leucovorin," she said.

"That's the vitamin B stuff that is supposed to help out the chemo, right?"

"Right," she said.

"Will it hurt?"

"Nope. Not at all. Feels just like a normal IV," she said.

She plugged the long, clear rubber tube attached to the leucovorin IV bag into the blue, pinky-sized rubber nub hanging from my forearm and pushed a few buttons on the *Star Wars* device. "I'll be back in 30 minutes to give you the 5-FU."

As the minutes ticked by, Mom and I chatted, and my stomach became queasy. Was it because I hadn't eaten breakfast or was it the leucovorin? I ate the bagel, which helped settle my stomach a little.

At the 30-minute mark, the *Star Wars* box beeped. My nurse appeared, pushed a few buttons to stop the beeping and sat down next to me with a large syringe.

"This is the chemo," she said.

"5-FU?"

"Yup."

"Will this one hurt?" I asked.

"Nope, although I've heard that some people experience a bit of a cold sensation in their arm as it goes in. How are you feeling?" She began pushing the syringe slowly into my IV line.

"OK. My stomach feels a bit weird, like I haven't eaten in a while."

"Someone usually comes around at about 11:30 to see if you'd like to have something brought up from the cafeteria. Try some juice in the meantime," she said, pointing to the bottle of cranberry juice that sat on a table next to me.

After 10 minutes, she pushed the last of the 5-FU into the IV line and pressed a few buttons on the *Star Wars* box again. "I'll be back in another 30 minutes," she said. "You have to finish the other half of the leucovorin."

I felt the chemo's iciness creeping up my arm and I was slightly more nauseated, as though I'd been in the backseat of a car for too long. There was a strange taste in my mouth too, like I was sucking on an empty spoon.

When the bag of leucovorin finished dripping into my body, my *Star Wars* box began to beep again and, right on schedule, my nurse returned and removed the IV line.

"You're all set," she said.

"That's it?" Mom asked. We had both been expecting it to take much longer, and I was sure I'd be throwing up on my way out the door, with clumps of hair in my hands.

"That's it. See you next week," the nurse said.

"That wasn't so bad," I said to Mom, as I rolled out the door with my skates still on. Altogether it had taken a little less than three hours.

"Don't forget what Dr. Martelo said. It's probably going to get worse. That was just your first treatment. He said each time they give you another treatment, the concentration of chemo in your body will go up."

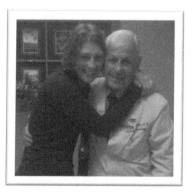

Me and Dr. Martelo

A week later, after my blood was tested, the nurse sat down on a rolling stool in front of me.

"How has your week been?" she asked as she unwrapped a needle and prepared my arm for the IV.

"Fine," I said.

"That's good. OK, here we go." I cringed as she stuck the needle into my arm and slid it into the vein. "Molly, if you hate needles so much, why don't you talk to Dr. Martelo about getting a port put in?" she asked. "It would make this a bit easier."

"What's a port?" I asked.

"It's actually called a port-a-cath. It's a port that is placed under your skin that connects to a catheter, which is placed in a large vein near your heart."

"What does it do?" I asked.

"Well, it allows easier access for us, for starters. It's also easier on your veins and has a lower risk of infection. We would still need to stick you with needles, but it's less painful than the traditional way, which is what we're doing now." She nodded at the tape-job she had just finished on my arm. "We can usually take blood from it as well."

"How do they put it in?"

"It's a simple day surgery," she said.

"No way! I'm not having any more surgery! Not for anything!"

"It's simple," she said again, "and you would be able to keep it for the duration of your chemotherapy. It's worth it."

"I'm not getting a port," I snapped again. "I've already had enough surgery to last a lifetime and then some. There's no way I'm going through another one. Besides, I play ice hockey, and the last thing I want is to get hit with a puck in the port!"

"Whatever," she said, laughing and standing up to retrieve my bag of leucovorin.

Most weeks, someone came with me. Usually it was Mom, sometimes it was Dad or Kristina. Dad and I talked, but when Kristina came it was like a day at camp. We joked and played cards with a deck from Colorado that featured pictures of bare-chested cowboys.

"What's that stuff they're giving you?" Kristina would ask each time she saw me.

"5-FU!" I laughed.

"Hey, don't talk to me that way! Do you kiss your mother with that mouth?"

When I looked around the room, I felt guilty for smiling and laughing. I saw sad faces and hairless heads all around me. Sometimes I wanted to feel sorry for myself, but Rocky's voice was always there: "You're going to make it through this. You'll beat it because you're strong – you're Molly."

I was so grateful for those words, encouraging me to make a choice every single day.

11

MARIE

I met Marie during my first six-week cycle of chemo. During one of the rare times that I went to chemo alone, I happened to sit next to the frail, little woman while waiting in the main lobby for my blood test results.

"I'll never get used to the number of needle sticks you get at as cancer patient," I said to the little stranger beside me.

She laughed. "You're telling me." Her accent was beautiful.

"Where are you from?" I asked.

"Schroon Lake," she said. "It's about an hour north."

"Oh, so that explains the French accent," I laughed.

"Originally, I'm from Canada, near Montreal."

We chatted until the nurse called her name.

"It was nice speaking with you," she said sweetly.

"You too," I said, watching her fragile, yet very put-together frame disappear through the door and into the "chemo lobby." She seemed so strong and matter-of-fact, as though today was just another day.

I settled into my chair and watched the *Today* show on the big television with the other patients. After 35 minutes, I followed a nurse into the "chemo lobby," where I was surprised to find my new friend hooked to an IV and a blue box.

"Is this seat taken?" I asked, nodding at the chair next to her.

"Oh, please join me," she said. "My name is Marie."

"I'm Molly."

"Awfully young to be here, aren't you?"

"That's what I've been told."

"Do you mind if I ask what kind of cancer?"

"Not at all. It's colon," I said, twisting my face.

"Me too," she said with a grin. She was probably at least three times my age, but in that moment, we became sisters.

"Hey, Moll," the nurse said. "Your counts look good, so we're just going to start your treatment."

"Great," I said, half joking.

"How was your week? Any trouble?"

"No, everything seems fine." I kept the constant diarrhea to myself, assuming it was from the surgery.

"I see you met Marie," the nurse said. She tapped the inside of my arm expertly with two fingers to find a good vein, which was getting harder to come by with each treatment. "She's a good lady to have around. Always smiling, but don't let her fool you. She's a tough one!"

The nurse pulled off the plastic top, exposing the needle and smiled at Marie. "Ready?" she asked, looking back at me.

"Errrrrr." I gritted my teeth and looked away.

"Molly, you should get a port," Marie said.

"I told you so," my nurse laughed.

"You have a port?" I asked. As I looked at Marie, I now noticed that her IV line didn't stop at her arm like mine. Instead, the long, clear plastic tubing snaked between two buttons of her shirt and then disappeared underneath.

"Yes," she said.

"Does it hurt?" I didn't want to offend her, but I was curious. She was the first person I knew with a port.

"No. Not at all."

"What about the surgery to put it in?" I asked.

"I think normally you have day surgery, but my surgeon put it in while I was in my last colon surgery. It's been wonderful. The only time I really know it's there is when I get treatment or when I have to flush it." I wasn't convinced, and quickly changed the subject.

"How are you feeling?" I asked.

"I have my good days and my bad. Today, I feel great. I had a big breakfast this morning on the way to treatment. I love a big breakfast. Omelet and sausage. Mmmm." I laughed at the sweet little woman with the delicate French accent, talking about eating a big breakfast.

"Are you on 5-FU too?" I asked.

"I used to be, but my side effects were pretty bad, so my doctor switched me."

"What happened?"

"The bottoms of my feet fell off in the shower one day."

"*What?*" I couldn't tell if she was kidding.

"I was on 5-FU and one day my feet just started to burn. It got worse and worse until finally I was in the shower and I just watched as layers of my skin begin peeling off. Then I had open sores that covered the bottoms of my feet. It's called Hand-Foot Syndrome and it's one of the possible side effects of 5-FU."

I was horrified.

"It was awful," she continued, "and that's when my doctor took me off the 5-FU and told me it was time to try something new." I secretly made a mental note to call Dr. Martelo immediately if I felt even the slightest bit of itching on my feet.

My mental vision of Marie's feet was interrupted by the beeping of her electric box.

"Guess I'm all done," Marie said. "Thank you so much for keeping me company.

"Are you kidding?" I asked as her nurse began to unhook her. "Thank *you*. And Marie, can I ask you something before you go?"

"Sure." She turned back to look at me.

"How long have you had colon cancer?"

"Four years and counting," she said with a smile. "I hope to see you again next week."

As I watched her walk away, I wondered how she could still be smiling after fighting colon cancer for so long.

That afternoon, I went home and lay in bed with that taste of metal in my mouth and a chemo hangover. Mom sat on the edge of my bed, running her fingers through my hair and rubbing my arm, just like she always had when I was a kid. I felt lucky to be home with her taking care of me like she did if I was sick during elementary school. What would have happened if I had stayed in Colorado and did chemo? With my face pressed into my pillow, I silently thanked Mom and Dad.

"Sorry I couldn't go to treatment with you today," Mom said.

"That's OK," I said. "I met a really nice lady."

"Another patient?"

"Yup. Colon cancer. We sat together during treatment."

"Was she your age?" Mom looked confused.

"Of course not." I laughed. "No one there is my age. I really liked her though."

"How are you feeling? Are you hungry?" she asked.

"I'm a little hungry, but my stomach is still pretty queasy."

"Maybe something light would help. What would you like?" she asked.

"I don't know."

"Soup?"

"No."

"A sandwich?"

"No."

"Yogurt?"

"No."

"Ice Cream?"

"Nothing dairy," I said, nearly gagging on the words. "Even ice cream sounds gross to me. I'm sorry I'm being so difficult, Mom."

"It's OK. What about some spaghetti?"

"Spaghetti sauce doesn't sound very good to me right now either."

"OK. Spaghetti, no sauce and some Parmesan cheese?"

"That might work."

"What about something to drink?" she asked.

"Is there any more of that grape Gatorade?"

"Sure is. I'll bring it up in just a few minutes."

As I drifted into sleep, I couldn't stop thinking about Marie. Cancer was so cruel.

For the next few weeks, I sat with Marie and took my chemo. I learned that she had a son who was a few years older than I was, and a sweet husband who drove her to chemo but always waited in the main lobby because he didn't like hospitals and was afraid to come into the room while she was undergoing her treatment. She had been a French teacher at Schroon Lake Central School, loved kids, and had a weak spot for big breakfasts and scratch-off Lotto tickets.

Marie was an incredible bright spot in a room that lacked happiness. She always smiled and spoke with all the patients, doctors and nurses around her, spreading her love. Just sitting next to her made my day better.

When it came to treatment, Marie was a great source of knowledge and that reinforced my confidence in my own outcome. She kept a chemo diary. Each day, she would write in her little red notebook what she ate or didn't eat, how she felt, when she vomited or had a case of diarrhea and how her energy level was. I was in awe of her dedication to that journal. Her diary helped her and helped her doctor better understand his patients.

We were completely different people with completely different lives, brought together by one stupid disease, but I was grateful for each day that I got to spend with Marie.

At the end of April, after my first four weeks of chemotherapy, I got a two-week break and finally visited my big brother at flight school in Florida. Dr. Martelo explained that during my break I would likely feel pretty good since some of the chemo would be leaving my body. He was right. I spent much of the break on my in-line skates with a hockey stick and tennis ball or relaxing by the pool.

My goal in Florida was to forget the world that awaited me at home. I wanted to forget about chemo and doctors and needles and my queasy stomach, but the more I tried to forget about it, the more I thought about Marie. I missed her while I was gone and wondered what she was doing during her two weeks off.

While walking on the beach alone one afternoon, it hit me hard. I was doing something that Marie might never get the chance to do again. She might never again see the ocean or smell the salty air and feel the warm sand between her toes. It wasn't fair. Why was such a beautiful person fighting an endless battle with colon cancer? Had God thrown a dart and she was the one it happened to hit?

As I walked down the beach something shiny caught my eye. I looked toward the water and there, where the waves were receding, I saw the most perfect, shiny, white shell. I jogged over and picked it up before the next wave could steal it away from me. It would be the perfect gift for Marie.

That night, at Rob's apartment, I wrote a message to Marie in marker on the inside of the shell. "Marie. You are my inspiration. Thank you for being my friend. Love, Molly."

When I arrived at the cancer center for my second round of chemotherapy, I found Marie, gave her a big hug, and handed her the shell.

"You brought this for me?" She laughed but had tears in her eyes.

Marie reached into her purse and handed me a small wad of tissue paper. Inside the paper, I found a beautiful, hand-painted brooch in the shape of a bird, black with a reddish-orange mark on its wing.

"I was thinking of you too," she said laughing. "I was at a craft show last week. When I saw it, I immediately thought of you and your spirit, just like a bird."

"Thank you so much," I said, hugging her again.

As treatment wore on and the side effects from chemo got worse, I stopped skating to the cancer center. On Monday mornings, I woke up nauseated just thinking about chemo.

Each week was nearly identical to the last, and I was becoming a seasoned chemo veteran, and comfortable enough to go alone. Once a week for four weeks I would stroll into the hospital, have blood taken, and then head into the "chemo lobby" with Marie and the other patients.

Dr. Martelo began sitting with me for a few minutes before each treatment, quizzing me on how I was feeling. My veins had turned a strange shade of orangey-brown, and even though I switched arms each week to combat overuse, it was becoming harder and harder for the nurse to insert the needle.

At the end of my three hours at the cancer center I usually went home and spent the rest of the day in bed, and sometimes most of Tuesday too. I felt weak, sleepy and queasy. My whole body ached. I was so tired, but I had trouble sleeping. Sometimes I cried for hours. The more chemo that went into my body, the more the metallic taste in my mouth increased. The nausea usually lessened when I ate but it was difficult to find anything that tasted good. I wouldn't touch things that I normally loved, like yogurt and ice cream. Grapes, Popsicles and pasta with only

Parmesan cheese became my staples, and I washed them down with purple Gatorade.

By Wednesday I usually perked up enough to play ice hockey at night with a local men's league. Other than seeing Marie, it was the one thing I looked forward to each week, and my only true escape from reality. When I was on the ice, I didn't think about what was happening to me off the ice, unless someone asked me about it, which wasn't often. I was the only woman, and as the weeks wore on, I found it harder and harder to keep up with the guys. Of course, just as I did in Colorado, I blamed myself for slowing down. I was lazy and wasn't in good enough shape. Maybe I wasn't drinking enough water, or I wasn't practicing enough. Never once did I blame it on the chemotherapy, even though each Monday morning, Dr. Martelo reminded me that the chemo in my system was increasing and soon I would have to take it easy.

One afternoon in July, while on my second two-week break from chemo, I stood in the kitchen with Mom and Dad, helping to make lunch.

"Daddy?" I said with the sweet voice of a 23-year-old daughter who was about to ask for something.

"Mokins?" he mimicked my high pitch while putting his silly twist on the nickname my friends all used.

"I miss my friends in Colorado," I continued, spreading tuna salad onto a slice of bread. "Can I have a frequent flier ticket to fly back and visit?"

"Get a job," he grumbled.

"Please, Dad? I really want to go back."

"What makes you think I have any tickets?" he asked, but I knew better. My father had traveled for work for as long as I could remember and had what I believed to be an endless supply of tickets available.

"Please, Daddy?" I used the best little girl voice I could muster. He usually couldn't resist.

"You just went to Florida to visit your brother a month ago. You can hang around with us *old* people a little bit longer."

"Pleeeeeeeease?" I begged, one last time.

"Why do you think you should be jetting off to Colorado while the rest of us are slaving away here?" His teasing was annoying. I hated when he had the upper hand.

"Fine," I said, feigning anger. "I'll just skate back, then." Mom looked up, wide-eyed, from the tomatoes she was cutting.

"Fine," he mumbled back. We were so alike and picked on each other like brother and sister, rather than father and daughter. Of course, we also both had to have the last word.

I stuck my tongue out at him, stormed out onto the porch, plopped down in a wicker chair and stared into the clouds. I watched a bird land in a tree and then take off again, flying out of sight. "Skate back," I said to myself, laughing out loud, but as though on cue, something clicked. I was overcome with excitement and purpose. People biked across the country for a cause all the time. Why couldn't I skate? The grin on my face widened. I could raise money, but more importantly, I could raise awareness of colon cancer in young people. The more people I told about my own cancer, the better and stronger I felt, as though I owned it instead of it owning me. If I skated halfway across the country, I could tell my story to anyone who would listen and prove that it wasn't just men over the age of 50 who were being diagnosed with the disease. Maybe when someone saw me, they would get screened or realize that it could happen to anyone. Maybe some college kid with unexplained symptoms would hear my story and push their doctor to give them a colonoscopy so they wouldn't have to go through the same hell that I did.

No matter what, at the end of the road I'd get to see my friends in Colorado. It was perfect!

But then Rocky flashed through my mind. What if he thought it was dumb? I would tell him first. His reaction would determine whether I did it or not.

That evening, after thinking about the trip all day, I called Rocky.

"Hello?" Even with just one word, the Boston accent came through.

"Hey, Rock."

"Hey, Moll! How are ya?" he asked excitedly.

"I'm great. You?"

"Neva betta!" he exclaimed. "So, what's up?"

"I think I have some news."

"You *think* you have some news? What is that?" he asked.

"Well, here's the thing," I began.

"There's always a thing," he interrupted, and I found myself giggling nervously and hoping he wouldn't laugh at me.

"Rock, I think I'm going to in-line skate back to Colorado to raise money and awareness of colon cancer."

There was a long pause.

"Are you *serious?*" he finally asked.

"I think so."

"That is *awesome!*" he exclaimed.

That was all I needed to hear. I *really was* going to skate back to Colorado.

When I arrived at the cancer center for treatment number one of my third cycle, I was a new woman with a purpose.

"Dr. Martelo, I have news," I announced as he sat down to ask his all-too-familiar list of questions. "During my chemo break I decided I wanted to do something crazy, to help raise awareness of colon cancer."

"OK," he said calmly. "Anything in particular?"

"It's pretty big." I waited for a reaction but got none. "You know how I'm always telling you that I play hockey and I love to skate?"

"Yes."

"Well," I stalled. He would probably think it was crazy. I hoped he wouldn't try to talk me out of it. "I've decided that I'm going to in-line skate to Greeley, Colorado to raise money and awareness of colon cancer.

"That's nice," he said. "Why Greeley? Didn't you go to school in Fort Collins?"

That was it? How was he not jumping out of his seat?

"Yes," I laughed, "but my friend Brad owns a roller hockey rink in Greeley. He said he would host a benefit tournament when I get there."

"Oh. And what are you going to call this skate?"

"Aimee came up with the perfect name last week – Rolling to Recovery!"

"That's wonderful, Molly." His voice never rose. "Now, speaking of Aimee, she is a wonderful young lady. Is your brother ever going to marry her?"

I should have known better. Dr. Martelo, somewhat like my father, was a hard man to impress.

"I hope so," I said, laughing.

"Good morning, Molly," the nurse said, as she approached with my IV. "How are you feeling?"

"Great, thanks. Have you seen Marie yet today?"

"She called this morning. Said she wasn't feeling well and asked if she could have a week off. She'll be back next week though."

"Oh." Suddenly, my excitement for Rolling to Recovery was smashed.

"So, what's the gossip that you were talking to Dr. Martelo about?" she joked.

"You're not going to believe this one," Mom said.

"Um, I think I'm going to in-line skate to Colorado next summer to raise money and awareness of colon cancer."

"Wow, Molly! That's fantastic!"

"Thanks," I said, but I was distracted. I wanted to share my news with Marie. She would have been so excited.

That afternoon, I went home and lay in bed. I had only had one treatment without Marie, but all I wanted to do was cry. Instead, I decided to call Rocky.

"Hellooooo?"

"Rock?"

"Yes, Swan?" he said.

"How are you?" I asked.

"I'm fine, but the *real* question is, how are *you?*"

"I'm OK," I said. "I had another treatment today."

"Oh, yeah?" he said, a little bit more serious. "How do ya feel?"

"Rock," I began, "I'm honestly so tired that I can't even sleep and my eyes just hurt. My whole body hurts, but there's no real place to point at that hurts."

"Moll," he interrupted. "Hold on. I have to tell you something." He was serious. "I was out the other night."

"Yeah?"

"And this termite walked into the bar."

"You're an idiot," I said laughing.

"And he said, 'is the bah-*tenda* here?'"

Rocky wasn't going to let me feel sorry for myself, and he would never know what that meant during a time in my life when I needed someone to make sure I chose *strong* every single time.

"I'm sorry, Moll," he said sympathetically, "but just think of how bad you'll feel around this time next year, skating across Nebraska in 115-degree heat."

"Thank you, Rock. You just made my day."

Over the next few days, I began telling everyone about my little trip on wheels. The more people I told about Rolling to Recovery, the less likely I was to back out. Or at least that's what I told myself. Besides, the idea didn't seem so crazy anymore since I loved skating so much. I was going to tell the world about my colon, and hopefully I could save someone from going through what Marie and I were going through.

When I arrived for treatment the following Monday, I immediately found the nurse. "Have you seen Marie?" I asked.

"She's getting her treatment in a private room today, Molly."

That wasn't like Marie. She liked to be with people; smiling, laughing and joking. "Would you please tell her that I'm worried about her and give her a hug for me?"

"She'll be happy to know that you're thinking of her," she said, and began my IV drip of leucovorin.

A few minutes later, I was greeted by a soft-spoken woman with a warm smile. "Molly?" she asked.

"Yes?"

"I'm Connie, from the American Cancer Society. Dr. Martelo called and told me about your idea to skate across the country," she said. "I think it's wonderful. He mentioned that you might like to donate some of the money to the American Cancer Society. Is that right?" she asked.

"Yes," I replied.

"Well, I just wanted to drop by and introduce myself and let you know that if you need anything, you can call me."

"That's really nice," I said, somewhat surprised. So far, everyone had liked my idea, but no one had volunteered to help.

"I brought you some envelopes so you can go door to door to collect money," she said. I nearly choked. I had absolutely no intention of going door to door. I had been thinking more along the lines of an interview on the *Late Show with David Letterman*.

"Thank you," I said, and took the envelopes, knowing that I would probably never use them.

"Envelopes?" I said to Mom, once the woman was out of earshot.

"Molly, she meant well."

"*Envelopes?*"

At my next chemo, after having my blood drawn, I looked for my nurse again. "Marie?" I asked.

"She's not feeling well again this week, Molly. She's in a private room."

"May I go and see her?"

"Follow me," she said. We walked down the corridor and stopped in front of a half open door. The nurse knocked lightly and pushed the door in.

"Marie?" she said softly.

Inside the room, Marie sat alone in a chair with her hands folded on her lap. She didn't wear any makeup and her hair was somewhat tousled, which was completely out of character. She looked up slowly when the nurse called her name.

"Hi, Marie, how are you?" I said softly. I pretended not to notice how tired she looked, but I was worried.

"I'm not feeling very well, Molly. I've had a bad week."

"You mean you didn't win any scratch-offs this week?" I tried to make a joke, and she laughed for a moment, but her laughter quickly turned to tears. I'd never seen her cry before. This was Marie, the adorable woman who always had a smile on her face and would never give up. I sat in the chair next to hers and put my arm around her.

"I was in for some tests earlier this week. I'm here to get the results and I just know they're not going to be good."

There was a soft tapping at the door and when it opened again, her doctor walked in followed closely by her husband. I gave her a hug and a kiss on the cheek. "It's going to be OK," I said as I left the room. "I love you."

I awoke to a soft tapping on my shoulder. I had dozed off in my chair during treatment. Shaking off the sleep, I slowly turned to see Marie with tears streaming down her soft cheeks.

"I'm terminal," she choked. "He has given me three months."

Her husband held her tightly as they walked away. I was devastated. I couldn't speak. This couldn't be happening to Marie. She was so strong and such a fighter.

Mom held my hand and we cried together through the rest of my treatment. At home, I got into bed and cried for most of the rest of the day. I just couldn't understand. This was Marie. She'd been my shining hope and was supposed to be one of the lucky ones. She had to be.

I lay in bed with my tears and wrote her a letter. I told her she was amazing and how much she inspired me. I told her that she gave me the courage to fight my own cancer. I told her about Rolling to Recovery and asked for her permission to dedicate it to her. Then I told her I loved her.

12

A NEW RUSSIAN FRIEND

🌢

O n Wednesday, I was still thinking about Marie, but needed to get out of *my* reality, so I went to my hockey game. I still felt drained from Monday's chemo and all the news that had come with it.

I suited up, and while waiting for the Zamboni to clean the ice, I found myself standing next to the handsome Russian who played in the league.

"Will you go out with everyone tonight?" he asked with a heavy accent.

"I don't know," I said. "I'm not a big partier, and I'm not supposed to drink anyway."

We'd only spoken once, a few weeks before when he apologized for checking me into the boards. As I lay on the ice and he looked down at me, his eyes had widened with surprise. I watched him process the fact that there was a girl playing ice hockey *and* that he had just hit her. "I'm sorry," he had said, offering me a hand. I was irate, of course. He would never have apologized if he had hit a man.

I thought everyone in the league knew I was a cancer patient, but when I hesitated on the drinks, he looked confused, and I felt awkward. When was the right time to tell someone I had cancer? I didn't want the whole conversation to be about it, but also didn't want it to look like I was hiding something. "I'm on chemotherapy," I blurted out. "I have colon cancer."

Again, his eyes widened, and without another word, my handsome new Russian friend turned, stepped onto the ice and skated away.

After the game, I joined the guys at the local Irish pub, hoping that Sergei, the handsome Russian, would show up for a drink. When I saw him walking up the sidewalk to our table on the outdoor patio, my heart began to beat a little faster. He took a seat across from me and we smiled back and forth, I with my water and he with his beer. Sergei had short, dark hair and big, beautiful eyes that smiled when he smiled. He wasn't much taller than me and looked about 18, but before he arrived, I found out from a few of my teammates that he was actually a few months older than me.

One by one, our teammates left, and soon it was just the two of us. I asked silly questions, just to keep him at the table. I learned that he was from Moscow and had been in the United States for two years, working in online banking. His parents were in Russia and his older brother and sister-in-law lived in Toronto. Sergei had recently gone sky-diving to celebrate his 24th birthday.

Playing hockey was the only thing that took my mind off of cancer, but now, as we talked and I looked into his eyes, I forgot all about it even without being on the ice.

How long have you been playing hockey?" I asked.

"I played in most of my childhood but stopped for a while when I was older. I just started playing again when I moved to United States. What about you?"

Because of his thick accent, I had trouble understanding, and I had to ask him to repeat what he said. "I used to figure skate when I was little, not competitively or anything, but that's where I first learned to skate. Then I roller-skated and in-line skated when that became popular, but I didn't start playing hockey until I was about 19 and living in Colorado."

"I've never seen a girl play hockey before," he said.

"Really? There were lots of us in Colorado. Did you know that because the U.S. Women's Ice Hockey Team won the gold medal at the Olympics in Nagano in '98, women's ice hockey is the fastest growing sport in the U.S. today?" I felt that I had to defend my sport.

"Why do you like hockey?" he asked.

"It's fun."

"But girls aren't supposed to like to play sports," he said.

"Why do you like hockey?" I interrupted, slightly offended.

"Because it's fun, but I'm a guy."

I could see that I had my work cut out for me.

Two days later, the phone rang, and Mom answered.

"It's the Russian guy," she whispered, handing me the phone.

"Hi, Molly. This is Sergei." I absolutely loved the way he said my name.

"Hi," I said, surprised to hear from him.

"Would you like to get together?"

"Um, sure," I said, trying to hide my excitement. "What would you like to do?"

"Do you play tennis?"

"I haven't played in a long time," I laughed, "but I'd love to!" I gave him directions to my parent's house and hung up the phone, giggling like an eight-year-old who just unwrapped a Barbie doll at Christmas.

When he arrived, Dad had to pull the "This-Is-My-Daughter-And-I-Own-A-Gun" routine, but Sergei didn't seem to mind. Maybe meeting parents wasn't such a big deal in Russia.

We played tennis for an hour or so at the YMCA's outdoor court, then he asked if he could take me to dinner. It was nice to actually be asked out. "Going out for a beer" had been the dating ritual in my Colorado college town.

As we chatted over lasagna and Cabernet, I tried to convince Sergei that girls and women could and should be allowed to do just about anything they wanted, including playing hockey.

Eventually, he asked me about the cancer. I told him about Colorado, my surgery and the trip to Dana-Farber where I'd had my first lobster. I told him about chemotherapy and Dr. Martelo and all the nurses. I told him about Marie. I probably told him too much, but it seemed like he wanted to hear it all. So, I just kept going, and he kept listening.

As we drove home that night, I really wanted to reach over and hold his hand. But fearing rejection, I didn't do it.

"Oh! Eleven, eleven," I said excitedly, breaking the silence in the car.

"What?" he asked.

"The time," I said, gesturing to the clock on his dashboard. "It's eleven, eleven. You're supposed to make a wish."

"Really? OK. What did you wish for?"

"I can't tell you," I said, laughing. "If I tell you, it won't come true."

"You're a silly girl," he said. When the car stopped at a red light, as if he was reading my mind, he put his hand on the back of my neck and ran his fingers gently through my hair. It was a subtle but caring gesture. A smile crept across my face. I had finally found something other than hockey that could make me forget about that other world I lived in. Just for a moment, I let go of cancer.

On Monday morning, I forced myself out of my Russian dreamland and back into reality. As I arrived at the cancer center, already nauseated, I was anxious for any news about Marie. I was terrified for her and felt guilty that her outcome would not be as lucky as mine. I'd had a fun-filled weekend, thinking about nothing but Sergei, when I should have been thinking about her.

"Has anyone heard from Marie?" I asked my nurse.

"She's in room seven," she said with a wink. "She'd love to see you."

I was sure I would find Marie in tears and gasping for breath, but instead she was looking as beautiful as ever and grinning as though she'd just scratched off the winning number.

I ran into the room and gave her a big hug. "I'm so glad to see you. What are you doing here?"

"I'm getting my treatment, Silly," she said. "I've decided that I'm going to fight." That was Marie. She was a petite kitten and a fierce tiger at the same time, and she was leading me by example. She had been fighting the battle for over four years with dignity and beauty, never complaining even though she knew that the outcome probably wouldn't be in her favor. She really was my hero.

"So, how have you been?" she asked.

"OK. I've been feeling pretty good and the chemo isn't..."

"That's not what I want to talk about," she interrupted. "How have *you* been?"

I beamed, thinking about my new Russian boyfriend. "I met a boy."

"*That's* what I want to talk about," she said. "What's his name?"

"Sergei. He's from Russia."

"And where did you meet him?"

"At hockey last week." It was the first time that Marie and I had really had a conversation about anything unrelated to cancer --- and it was nice.

"Is he handsome?"

"Yup," I said.

"Molly, we've got your treatment ready," my nurse said, popping her head into the room.

"Thank you. I'll be right there. Sorry, Marie. Apparently, girl talk is over. Duty calls."

"Thanks for worrying about me," she said.

"Thanks for being you," I answered back, kissing her on the cheek.

As my nurse started my IV and the lights on the blue box began to flash, I thought about Marie. I couldn't feel sorry for myself anymore. When I looked at the people who sat around me in the "chemo lobby," the truth was obvious. I still had my hair. I still smiled, and I still played hockey once a week. My prognosis was good. I would finish my chemo and live the rest of my life without needles and blood tests. I would eventually outgrow the constant checkups, but many of the other patients would continue their chemo. They would live the rest of their lives around their treatments.

By the time my fourth and final round of chemotherapy came, the side effects were finally catching me. Although I had never thrown up, the nausea was worse than ever, and I was tired most of the time.

Dr. Martelo finally put his foot down. "Molly, your body is dealing with a powerful drug, and the concentration is getting extremely high. You need to get as much rest as you can for the last cycle."

"No more hockey?" I asked.

"No more hockey," he said.

I was almost relieved. It was harder and harder to keep up with the guys, but I hadn't allowed myself any excuses, even though it was hurting my confidence on the ice.

"I'm still allowed to go and watch, right?"

"You can go and watch," he said.

"I have a new boyfriend. He's on the team, you know."

"Lots of bed rest," he repeated.

"Yes, sir."

Sergei and I began spending most of our free time together. We played tennis when I had the energy and went out for dinner and to movies. On hockey nights, I sat in the stands watching, secretly happy to have a doctor's note that kept me off the ice. On days when I wasn't feeling well, we would curl up together in his tiny apartment and watch a movie.

One night, he stroked my hair and whispered a few Russian words into my ear.

"What does that mean, Sergei?"

"It means 'I love you,'" he said.

Sergei was smart and mature, caring and gentle. My family and friends loved him. As I got to know him, I was surprised to find that the chauvinistic European attitude he had revealed when he told me that women shouldn't play hockey wasn't really chauvinistic at all. In Russia, he was taught that women should be taken care of. This made me feel soft and feminine, which didn't come naturally to my tomboyish character.

While Sergei was growing up in Moscow and learning to treat women like delicate flowers, I was playing in the dirt in upstate New York. As a kid, my chores were taking out the garbage and mowing the lawn, as well as setting and clearing the table. Dad bought me hammers for Christmas. That was his way of telling me that I should never rely on anyone else to get things done. I could and *should* be able to do anything.

Slowly, over time, I learned to put my cynicism aside and accept Sergei's sweet and endearing gestures as his desire to take care of me, not to make me feel weak. I loved the way he always held my hand or put his arm around me. I was falling in love.

One Monday morning, Sergei joined me at chemo, a stack of movies in his hands. I was nauseated when I woke up that morning and asked to receive my treatment in a private room.

"Is this a *date*?" my nurse teased, as she put in my IV line. "Did you bring a *date* to chemo?"

"I guess so," I said, blushing.

She laughed. "Molly, you're the only person I know that would bring a *date* to chemo." I laughed and looked at Sergei, who was shyly ignoring us.

As soon as my IV was hooked up, Sergei started playing the movie, but soon we were both asleep in the small hospital bed.

I awoke to feel the nurse pushing the 5-FU into my IV line and Sergei's arms wrapped tightly around me. She winked at me and smiled. Sergei and I stayed like that for the rest of my treatment. I don't know if he did it because he thought I was scared and wanted me to feel safe or if he was the one who was scared, but I didn't want to ever lose the loving feeling of his arms around me. I looked at the clock. *Eleven, eleven. Make a wish.* I looked at Sergei and wished that he would be the man I would marry.

A few weeks later, I received a letter from the Empire State Games Selection Committee. It was an application to try out for the Adirondack Women's Ice Hockey Team, which would play in a six-team, round-robin tournament at the Empire State Games in Lake Placid in mid-February. Tryouts were on December 5, just under two months after I was set to finish chemo.

I picked up the phone and called Rocky.

"I was just invited to try out for a spot in the Empire State Games!" I said.

"Congratulations, Swan! What are ya talking about?"

"Sorry," I laughed. "Empire State Games – they are sort of like the New York State Olympics for amateurs," I said.

"So, what are ya callin' me for?"

"I don't know. I guess I'm not sure that I'll be able to make the team."

"Molly, what's 'a matta with ya'?"

"Rock, I've been off the ice. My doctor hasn't been letting me play."

"So?"

"I'm really out of shape."

"So?" I was hearing exactly what he heard -- excuses.

"Molly, ya don't need to hear me say it, but what's the worst thing that could happen?"

"I don't make the team."

"So, what's the big deal? Then you're right back where ya started, which isn't a bad place to be, ya know?"

"But what if I don't?"

"Hey, it's free ice time, and that's not easy to come by." I laughed. "Molly, all I've ever wanted to do is play professional hockey. When I get out of the military my girlfriend is gonna kill me for it, but I have to try, or I'll regret it for the rest of my life. Go for it!"

I knew he was right. "Thanks, Rock," I said.

"Just 'rememba' one thing," he said.

"Not the termite," I begged.

"No, seriously," he said. "Every girl is there because they want *your* spot on the team. Be friendly in the locker room, but *not* on the ice. That's *your* spot."

I filled out the form and mailed it back.

When I arrived at the cancer center for my final dose of chemotherapy, I couldn't will my white blood count to stay up anymore, and Dr. Martelo said I couldn't get my treatment.

"Please," I begged. "I promise not to leave the house all week."

"Molly, I know you want to finish, but if something goes wrong, you'll end up in the hospital. I cannot give you your treatment this week."

I went home and cried and waited until the following Monday.

On Monday, October 11, 1999, nearly nine months after I had been diagnosed with colon cancer, I received my last chemotherapy treatment. There was nothing ceremonial about it. I would get a checkup in three months. That was it. I had gone to chemo every Monday for four weeks, then enjoyed two weeks off before the process started over again -- 16 treatments in all.

I went home relieved and a little sad, unsure of what would happen next. I got into bed, took a long nap, and dreamed about scoring the gold-medal-winning goal at the Olympics with the Women's U.S. Ice Hockey Team.

That evening, Sergei stopped by my parents' house on his way home from work.

"Congratulations, Baby!" he exclaimed with a wink and handed me a medium-sized brown paper bag.

I opened the bag and let out a yelp. A live lobster with beady eyes stared up at me. I hugged Sergei. I couldn't believe he remembered the story about my first lobster after the Dana-Farber visit. Then I grabbed a pot and started filling it with water.

The following week, Sergei and I boarded a plane to Orlando. He had never been to Florida, and I wanted to get cancer off my mind. We rented a convertible and spent two weeks traveling to Orlando, Daytona Beach, Key West and Miami.

"I think I know what I want to raise money for when I skate next summer," I said one afternoon while lying on the beach.

"I thought you already said that you were going to give it to the American Cancer Society," he said.

"Some of it," I replied, "but I want to give some to my cancer center. And I've been debating what to do with the last third. "I think I want to support young patients. They have a lot to deal with. Maybe they just want to forget it all and go away for a week, just like we're doing now."

When we returned to New York, there was a Christmas card waiting for me. Inside, I found a New York State Lottery Ticket. Written inside the top of the card in perfect cursive was the slogan "Hey – You never know!" and under that was a note.

Dear Molly,

I was thrilled to watch you on a special Channel 13 segment. Congratulations and keep up the good work! Wow...you're a celebrity now!

I'm very weak and still won't stop fighting this monster...

All my love,
Marie

I didn't have much time to prepare for the Empire State Games tryouts, but I hoped for the best. Then, on December 5, seven weeks after I finished chemo, Sergei and I headed north to Plattsburgh, about 100 miles away.

Marie's house was on the way, so we picked up some flowers and scratch-off tickets and dropped by for a quick visit. She looked tired and frail, but even in her pajamas, she was still beautiful and composed and, of course, excited about the scratch-off tickets. She fed us homemade meatball soup, then I kissed her goodbye and we were on the road again.

The tryout lasted three hours. We were on the ice for an hour and a half of drills, took a break while the Zamboni resurfaced the ice, then got back on for an hour and a half scrimmage. I was sure I wouldn't be able to keep up, but once my adrenaline got pumping, I forgot about any doubts I had and just gave my best. My skating was solid and, although I wasn't as fast or as fluid handling the puck as some of the other women, I held my own. At the end of the scrimmage, the coach told us to get dressed and meet him in the conference room.

"Thank you all for coming. Everyone did an excellent job," he said. "There's not a single one of you that I wouldn't like to have on my team." I played nervously with my necklace, the one Sarah had given me, while he looked around and met each set of eyes. "Unfortunately, I can only take 18 skaters, two goalies and two alternates. I have the list right here," he said, holding up his clipboard. "If I call your name, you've made the team."

He began calling off names, one by one. I couldn't remember ever being so nervous. As the list got longer and longer and I still hadn't heard my name, I was overcome with disappointment. But then, just as I was thinking about what Rocky said about the free ice time, I heard the coach call out "Molly McMaster." For a moment, I wasn't sure I had heard correctly, but my teammates were congratulating me. I had made the team! I was going to play in the 2000 Empire State Games. I looked over at Sergei. He gave me the thumbs up sign.

Just days after I made the team, Marie went into the hospital. My heart clenched when I visited her and saw how frail she was. She cried as she told me that she was waking up each morning and praying that God would take her that day. She asked me to pray for her to die, but I couldn't do it. Instead, I held my friend as she put her head on my shoulder and cried. It took everything I had not to cry too. I wanted to be strong for her.

Louise "Marie" Gaillardet succumbed to colon cancer on January 27, 2000, more than six months after the day her doctor had given her the horrible news.

I was heartbroken and angry and more driven than ever before. No matter what happened, the year 2000 was going to be my year. I was going to grab it, run with it and never look back.

PART III

MY FIGHT AGAINST CANCER

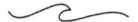

"Every accomplishment starts with the decision to try."

Gail Devers
Olympic Champion
Track and Field

13

POOR LITTLE GIRL WITH CANCER

Once they've survived cancer, people do things they never thought they could do. Many will give you the old cliché, "I'm going to live life to the fullest," and then rattle off a handful of bucket list items they've completed and others that they are planning to do. I guess that makes sense. It did for me. After colon cancer, I was ready to try anything. I felt *stronger* --- unafraid --- courageous. I told everyone that 2000 was going to be *my* year, but even I didn't realize what that might entail.

Before cancer, if I had made a list of things I would *never* do in my lifetime, entering a beauty pageant would have been in the top five. Then along came cancer, and somehow I let Sarah talk me into entering the local winter carnival pageant.

"Come on, Moll. If nothing else, it will get you some publicity for Rolling to Recovery," Sarah had argued one night.

"Alright, fine. But only if you go and watch the whole, hilarious thing."

"You're on!" she said.

A few weeks before the pageant, I had abdominal pain and generally was not feeling well, so Dr. Martelo ordered some tests. I put my lucky necklace on and went back to the hospital. The CT scan revealed some dark spots on my liver.

"You'll need an MRI," the doctor told me. The results from that test also showed something, so next it was a needle biopsy, scheduled the day before the pageant. When I went to the hospital, I was too nervous to think about the pageant and still didn't know what I'd be doing for the talent section. I was not a beauty queen. While the other girls were at the tanning salon and getting their hair and nails done, I was lying face down in the CT scan machine with an oversized needle stuck into my back. After the biopsy, I was wheeled into recovery, where I threw up from the anesthesia.

The day of the pageant, I was the first contestant to arrive at the hotel and I was armed with three sequined dresses, a small makeup case, my in-line skates, hockey gloves and a stick. I was determined to be different. The second woman to arrive lugged a large pink case, which I assumed could only be a tackle box for deep sea fishing.

"Hi," she said, dropping it on the floor and opening it to reveal a huge stash of makeup. There was my confirmation. I was in the *wrong* place. My little silver makeup palette was embarrassing, but I wasn't sure if that was because I lacked expertise in beautifying, or because she seemed so overzealous.

One by one, the women arrived and we busied ourselves with primping until it was time for the first segment of the pageant. Each woman was brought individually onto a stage in the hotel ballroom to answer a different question. As I waited for my name to be called, giggling nervously with the other women, one question perplexed me: "What is the one thing you would change about yourself and why?" I listened intently as the girl ahead of me answered the question, saying something about her facial imperfections.

What would I change? As I stood in line, preparing to do one of the most ridiculous things I'd ever done, I thought about my cancer and the chemo and the day before, when a black X was drawn in permanent marker on my back at the place where the biopsy needle would go. I still couldn't rub it off. I thought about Marie. As my name was called, I caught Sergei's eyes as he sat in the back of the room with Mom, Dad and Sarah. I was so lucky to have such a wonderful family and friends. I thought of how the stupid cancer had brought us closer together somehow. I smiled as I entered the ballroom and realized that there was nothing I would change. My life was perfect – it was mine – and I liked it just the way it was.

Now it was time to put my talent to the test. I changed into my old prom dress, a short, backless, sequined number and put on my in-line skates and stinky hockey gloves. Ridiculous or not, I was having fun. The second time I entered the ballroom, I was escorted by a Naval Cadet, who held his breath from the stench of my gloves. I laughed when I heard him gasp for air as he left my side.

I dropped a golf ball on the floor and skated around the room, whacking the ball as I told the audience and judges about myself, my hockey, and my colon cancer. I also apologized for the lack of ice. When I finished, I wasn't sure if the talent I had displayed was hockey or public speaking, but I had definitely left an impression.

There were only seven of us in the pageant, and I came in dead last, but I never felt even a hint of embarrassment. Surviving colon cancer was better than any crown, and sharing my story with the crowd while sporting a cocktail dress and hockey skates would definitely not be soon forgotten. As an athlete, I had learned how to accept defeat with grace and a smile.

A few days later, Dr. Martelo called with the results of the biopsy. The spots were benign. My cancer had *not* come back.

"I believe it's just fatty tissue," he said. I let out a sigh of relief. It was the first time I'd ever been excited about extra fat.

Two weeks later, I celebrated my 24th birthday and the first anniversary of my diagnosis. On that same weekend, I stepped onto the ice at the Lake Placid Olympic Center as a member of the Empire State Games Adirondack Women's Ice Hockey Team. The competition at the Games was the best I'd ever played with, and after four games in three days and almost exactly one year after my diagnosis, the Adirondack Team stepped off the ice with gold medals hanging around our necks. It was a victory for all of us, but a special one for me. My personal victory was my health, my life and proof that I would never be that poor little girl with cancer that I was so afraid of becoming.

As I came down from my cloud, it was time to prepare for the road ahead. I had just skated in the Empire State Games, but I was still in no shape to skate across the country. I kissed my hockey skates goodbye and put them into the closet, replacing them with my in-line skates. With February snow still on the ground, I began training at the local indoor roller skating rink and lifting weights at a gym. Preparing for Rolling to Recovery was my new job and I had to get into shape and beg for money and supplies for the trip.

Although I had no idea what I was doing, I sent out sponsorship letters and e-mails asking for money, skates, wheels, sports drinks, water and even an RV. For every 25 requests I sent out, I received 24 rejection letters. It was disappointing but at the same time, when I received a commitment, my spirit was rekindled and I took one more stride toward my goal.

"I reserved rollingtorecovery.com for you," Sergei said one evening.

"What for?" I asked.

"What do you mean, 'what for'?" You have to have a website!"

"Oh," I laughed. "But I don't know how to do any of that stuff."

"Relax. Just give me a few weeks."

Sergei spent every free moment working on it, and before I knew it, I had my own website that told my story and featured pictures, a map of my route from New York to Colorado and a guestbook.

"If you keep an online diary, people will be able to track your daily progress," he said. "There's even a place to donate."

I started getting emails and sign-ins on my guestbook from all over the country, and each day I answered every one with a personal message. People were actually finding out about my planned journey. Even with my ever-growing "to do" list, the excitement was overwhelming.

One day, there was an email from the friend of an old Colorado roommate. I didn't know him well, but I remembered that he looked like Patrick Roy, the goalie at the time for the Colorado Avalanche. He told me that his mother, Nancy, had been diagnosed with colon cancer. He gave me her email address, asking if I would send her a note, which I did. I didn't say much, just told her that I was thinking of her and if she needed a friend, to please stay in touch. And so began my first online friendship with another colon cancer patient.

Nancy reminded me a lot of Marie. They were about the same age and had both been diagnosed at a later stage. Just like Marie, Nancy was sweet and kind and turned out to be a wonderful email buddy, checking in a few times a week and always asking for the latest report on Rolling to Recovery.

Meanwhile, the Rolling to Recovery planning committee was meeting once a month in the main lobby of the cancer center. Little by little, my trip was becoming something big.

Late in the winter, Monaco Coach, a national manufacturer of recreational vehicles, agreed to loan us a 37-foot luxury motor coach for the summer, complete with two TVs. Mom had volunteered to drive it. We certainly wouldn't be roughing it.

"You're not my Mom on this trip," I said during one meeting as Mom scolded me for dropping cookie crumbs.

"Here we go," she laughed.

Shortly after that, someone in my guestbook said that they had read about me in *Mademoiselle* magazine. I had no idea how *Mademoiselle* heard about me, but I rushed out to buy a copy and found a two-line blurb at the bottom of an article about in-line skating for fitness: "Molly McMaster, 24, and a colon cancer survivor, will skate 2,000 miles in May to raise money to fight cancer. Check out www.rollingtorecovery.com."

"Look at this!" I squealed to the woman in front of me at the checkout. "That's me!"

On March 31, 2000, less than two months before I was scheduled to depart, the local pro-hockey team, the Adirondack IceHawks, held a Rolling to Recovery Night at one of their games. They donated $1,000 to Rolling to Recovery and gave me a table in the lobby of the Glens Falls Civic Center to educate people about colon cancer and tell them about Rolling to Recovery. The highlight of the night was a ceremonial puck drop at center ice just before the game began.

After both teams were on the ice and the national anthem was hitting its final notes, I stood with one of the front office employees in the pit, the place where the visiting team waits before they go on to the ice. Because Rolling to Recovery Night was a celebration of my in-line skate cross-country, I was wearing my hockey skates.

"It's just about time," he said to me, handing me an official game puck. I smiled and took the puck. Then the arena went dark. A lone spotlight seared through the blackness and landed at the door where I was to enter the ice.

"Ladies and gentlemen," the announcer said over the PA, "Please join me in welcoming Molly McMaster to the ice this evening to drop the IceHawks ceremonial puck!"

I stepped on to the ice and into the spotlight wearing black dress pants, a bright red shirt and a smile from ear to ear. As I glided toward center ice, the announcer continued.

"Molly is a colon cancer survivor who was diagnosed at just 23. This summer she'll in-line skate from Glens Falls to Greeley, Colorado to raise awareness of colon cancer." The crowd cheered as I arrived at center ice and shook hands with both team captains under the shining spotlight.

The two opposing players lined up on either side of the face-off dot, and I bent my knees and hunched over, holding the puck over the dot, ready to make the drop. I looked up at the visiting captain and back at the IceHawks captain. For a moment, I had a twinge of jealousy. They were living my dream. I would never get to play in the Olympics, or even in college, for that matter. My time had long since passed. I grinned and leaned over to the IceHawks captain.

"How about if *you* drop the puck and *I* take the faceoff," I said.

He laughed, but I felt like he was reading my mind.

"Sure," he said, handing me his gloves and stick and taking the puck from me. "My gloves are pretty gross."

"Ah, whatever. I'm sure mine are just as bad," I said as I slid my hands into what felt like a fresh batch of sludge.

Maybe not.

The crowd applauded, and I looked up at the Mohawk Valley Prowlers captain with a huge smile before taking what would probably be the only "professional" face-off of my lifetime. It felt *awesome.*

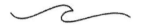

By May, word was really getting out about my trek.

Dear Molly:

Barbara Krogmann wrote me recently and shared with me what a role model you have been for the Glens Falls community. You sound like a truly amazing woman. Thank you for all of your efforts to raise awareness about colon cancer. I can't tell you how many touching personal stories people have shared with me. This type of cancer affects so many people and leaves such devastation in its wake. It is truly a national tragedy.

Please thank Barbara for sharing your personal story with me and for taking the time to write. And good luck with your rollerblading trip! My girls have been bugging me to learn how --- you might just be the inspiration I need!

Sincerely,
Katie Couric

Now there was no turning back. I would spend the summer on in-line skates in the blistering heat with Mom behind me, and we would tell my story to anyone who would listen. There had to be more young people out there like me, having symptoms and going to their doctors, but being told that they were only constipated. It would only be a matter of time before I found one. It didn't take long.

One afternoon, I was surprised by an email I found in my inbox.

Hi. My name is Amanda Sherwood Roberts and I'm 25 years old and a colon cancer survivor just like Molly. She is the first person that I have even heard of that is my age and has had colon cancer. Most everybody is older. I would really love to have the opportunity to speak with her and hear about her experience. I am a member and volunteer with the Colon Cancer Alliance.

Amanda Sherwood, Stage III
Little Rock, Arkansas

I stared at the screen in shock. Except for the oncologist I had seen in Boston, all the doctors and nurses had told me over and over again how impossible it was for me to have colon cancer at my age. Yet here was someone just like me. And she was also fighting for people to realize that it could happen to someone in their twenties.

I wrote back, asking her to forgive me for my brief response, and explaining that I was getting ready to skate to Colorado to raise awareness for our disease. *Our* disease. It was strange, not having to call it only *my* disease anymore. I told her I was so thankful to know that there was indeed someone out there, just like me, and asked if we could please keep in touch.

Dear Molly:

I had the privilege of meeting you Tuesday at the Channel 8 program. Your courage and giving spirit is something very special and amazing. Thank you for sharing your life and hope to others.

Best of luck on your journey. You will be the beacon of "light" for many in your travels.

The Emergency Care Center --- Laura Stebbins
** We hope you won't need anything in the first aid kit!

Accompanying the note was an "Emergency Care Center in a Box," a first aid kit the hospital put together for my road trip.

On the morning of Saturday, May 20, 2000, the day I started my journey, I got up early to meet a reporter from *The Post-Star*, my hometown newspaper. I munched on a bagel, loading up on carbs to fuel the first 21 miles of my journey. The reporter interviewed me in my parents' living room, on the same green couch where Dr. Thompson had removed my staples.

"Are you sure you'll finish?" the reporter asked. I laughed. It was a question I heard over and over again. No one seemed to understand that there was absolutely no doubt in my mind that I would finish. It had been one year, three months and one day since I was told that I had cancer. I had endured two surgeries, almost nine months of chemotherapy, and had lost a good friend to the disease. This was the easy part.

"Quitting is *not* an option," I said confidently.

I followed the reporter outside and was greeted by TV reporters and photographers plus friends and neighbors who had come to see me off. The sky was darkening, and as I sat on the porch, tightening my skates and posing for a news crew, Christian's parting words at Green Mountain College flashed through my mind. "I won't be surprised if you're back here within a year." But his voice, which had ached for so long in my ears, was only a whisper. I would skate through a thundering downpour to get back to Colorado, to get back to life before cancer and to prove Christian wrong.

14

ROLLING TO RECOVERY
THIS SIDE OF THE MISSISSIPPI

At 9:45 a.m., I hugged Dad and Sergei, waved goodbye to friends who had gathered to see me off, and gave a thumbs-up to Mom, behind the wheel of the RV, which we had affectionately begun calling the "Big Dog."

Light rain was falling as I rolled to the bottom of the driveway onto Garrison Road and followed the flashing lights of the police cruiser, which was flanked by two more officers on bicycles. Another cruiser fell in behind, and I was whisked to downtown Glens Falls for an official send-off at City Park.

A small crowd stood waiting when we arrived at the bandstand, and I rolled up the red carpet to meet the police chief, mayor, and many friends and town officials, who took turns offering their best wishes. Then the mayor stepped to the microphone to proclaim May 20, 2000 as

"Molly McMaster Day." He handed me the official proclamation and gave me a hug. Grandma sat in the crowd, and while I'll never be sure, I think I saw her wiping tears from her eyes.

The crowd began a countdown. "Ten. Nine. Eight." I gave my necklace an excited squeeze. "Three. Two. One!"

Before I knew it, I was skating south out of the city on U.S. Route 9, with a crowd of bicyclists and skaters in tow and the "Big Dog" following. Somewhere far off, on the horizon of my imagination, was Colorado.

The crowd braved the steady drizzle as we left Glens Falls, our elation overshadowing the dark and dreary skies. I had no doubt that I would keep putting one skate in front of the other all the way to Colorado, no matter what obstacles I encountered.

Each day presented a new challenge. The first three it was rain. On the fourth day, when we parted from the last of our friends just as the sun finally came out, I faced the hills of central New York State. A little more than an hour's drive from home on U.S. Route 20, they began small enough, teasing me as they rolled gently through farmers' fields, but soon they sloped steeper and stood taller, no longer hills but mountains that I would need to conquer one by one. On one of them, I couldn't even see the summit as I began my ascent and struggled for an hour to reach the top. On the way down, I needed to do a controlled slalom, crossing both lanes of the road. This pushed Mom's heart rate well above where it should have been, as she was supposed to be driving a leisurely, 10 miles per hour.

By the time I reached the bottom of one lumbering giant, my thighs burned and ached, but in front of me loomed another.

It didn't matter. This was nothing like what Marie had to go through. I was spending my days on skates, my absolute favorite place in the world. When we rolled into a new town, reporters and television crews met us and we shared the story of the young colon cancer survivor who was headed to the Wild West to show the world that the disease could happen to anyone. Every time my tale was told, there was a chance that someone out there would start a conversation they needed to have. I couldn't begin to imagine a better way to spend a summer.

The miles slowly ticked away. Mom and I took our first break, in the village of Tully, south of Syracuse, New York, to visit with cousins.

"Here, Trudie," cousin Karen said, after dinner, handing Mom two crumpled dollar bills. "We've been following the daily journal entries. The boys asked if they could donate their weekly allowance to Rolling to Recovery."

"That's so sweet," Mom said, fighting tears.

Rolling to Recovery had started as a joke – a way to go back to Colorado to visit friends. But at that moment, watching as Mom put the two dollars into an envelope, it struck me. Our journey wasn't just about visiting Colorado or raising awareness. It was giving hope to cancer patients and survivors, and it was also showing little boys and girls across the country that one person could truly make a difference.

"Good work, Mokins," Dad said one night on the phone. "230.3 miles down. 10 percent of the mileage is gone and 12 percent of the time!"

Eleven days into my trip, I received a second email from my new friend, Amanda.

Molly,

I was so excited to hear back from you. I know you are busy now, and I envy you for what you are doing. I would love to talk to you, if not in person, voice to voice would be great!

I was diagnosed in January of 1999 with Stage III colon cancer at age 24. At the time, my daughter was three and my son was four months old. It has been a long, hard road. I am now a member of the Colon Cancer Alliance (CCA) on the advocacy and administrative committees. I found CCA while searching for statistical information on younger people with colon cancer. I work for the Arkansas Secretary of State, so I'm trying to use my position here to help get support for colon cancer funding.

Anyway, good luck on your trek! I will keep you in my thoughts and prayers!

Amanda

Amanda had been diagnosed only one month before me. I slipped back into the memory of my own illness. Amanda was suffering in Little Rock while I was in the same misery in Colorado. What if we had connected with each other *before* cancer? And how was my cancer at stage II, but she was stage III?

I emailed her back right away.

The farther west we went, the brighter the sky became, and the hills settled down, becoming low and rolling and more fun. Once Mom and I settled into life on the road, we spent what little free time we had in the grocery store, to restock our food and see some different scenery. Our days were structured. We'd get up, have breakfast and call the local media. I would get dressed and skate for as long as the weather, or my body, would allow. When we finished for the day, I would write a journal entry.

Then we would find a local hotel that would allow us to use a phone line to connect to the internet and email my journal entry and any photos to Sergei to post on the website that night. Finally, we would find a clean and safe place to park the "Big Dog" for the night, which was never an easy task. We would make dinner and take showers. I would clean and rotate the wheels on my skates and then go to bed ready to greet the next day and do it all again.

Dad called one night, as Mom and I were beginning our nightly routine.

"Hey, Mokins."

"Dad! We just put the New York State map away! We're in Pennsylvania!" I proclaimed.

"Congratulations," Dad said, somewhat sternly. "Now get out the U.S. map."

I cringed as I unfolded the U.S. map and counted the states between us and Colorado, noting that they were bigger the farther west my finger moved. Nebraska would certainly destroy me. "Thanks, Dad," I said. He laughed. "You're a real buzzkill."

"Just putting it all into perspective for you," he joked.

But the next day was perfect. I caught my first tailwind on a flat road, and all three major Erie news networks tracked us down. The more people I told about my cancer, the more sense I was able to make of it, as though it happened to me for a reason. The media had become my vehicle, and I watched jaws drop when people heard the unbelievable story of the young woman diagnosed with colon cancer at just 23. I didn't fit the stereotypical face of colon cancer, and it was a picture I hoped they would never forget.

By the end of the day I'd logged 60.2 miles and skated into state number three, Ohio, Christian's home state.

I thought about calling him. A small part of me wanted him to see *me* --- see that I had beaten the wind, the hills and the rain and wasn't headed home anytime soon. I decided to email him.

A few days later, the rain came again, too much to go on, so Mom and I spent two nights with Dad's old college roommate. Phil set up photo shoots with two newspapers and arranged for a news crew to do a story the day before I would take on Cleveland.

It was nice to take a few days off from skating and just talk to the media and visit with Phil and his wife, but when the sun came back out, Mom and I were anxious to get back on the road. After the news crew left, we waved goodbye and I skated 21 miles to Mentor, just outside of Cleveland.

We called it a day when the wind picked up and the temperature started to fall. In the RV, we turned on the TV and caught the last few minutes of *The Oprah Winfrey Show*. Then we saw what we were waiting for.

"She's a vibrant, athletic, beautiful young woman." I zoomed across the screen wearing the same red pullover rain jacket that I still had on. "She's also had cancer." The screen changed and a bubbly, blonde anchorwoman appeared.

"Good afternoon. When you think of colon cancer, more often than not the picture you see is a middle-aged man, not a 23-year-old, normally healthy woman." Mom and I sat in stunned silence, neither of us expecting to be the lead story on the five o'clock news in Cleveland. "Molly McMaster *is* that woman. The cancer survivor is now in-line skating across the country, raising money and awareness about this deadly disease that can attack anyone. Our own Roosevelt Leftwich caught up with Molly and her mother outside of Cleveland this afternoon." The screen cut to the video they had taken earlier in the day.

"Good Golly, Miss Molly. You sure like to roll. So far Molly McMaster has rolled through three sets of wheels and over 450 miles in a celebration of life after cancer. Two years ago, this athletic college student had symptoms of the disease that most people associate with old men – colon cancer." Mom buzzed across the screen in the "Big Dog," chasing after me.

"I can't believe we just followed *Oprah*!" I said, talking over the reporter as he continued with some colon cancer statistics. "I wonder how many people just watched that?"

"A *lot*," Mom said. "A *lot* of people just learned about colon cancer."

That night I received a reply email from Christian. He didn't tell me if he had seen the news, just gave me his number and told me to call when I reached the Cleveland city limits. He would be working but would love to take a break and meet us to say hello.

The next morning, at an intersection near our starting point, a woman pulled to a screeching halt next to the "Big Dog" and rolled her window down.

"Where's the skater? Where's the skater?" she squealed.

"She's right here," Mom laughed, leaning back in the driver's seat so I could wave to her from the passenger side.

"I read about you on the front page of the paper this morning and saw you on TV! You rock! You're awesome!"

I had no idea who the stranger was, but she gave me the kick I needed to conquer Cleveland. As I laced up my skates, I felt invincible, like I could plow through 500 miles in blowing wind and rain if I had to.

An hour later, on the steps of the Rock and Roll Hall of Fame, I saw Christian approaching.

We exchanged greetings and hugged awkwardly. The sun was bright, but I took off my sunglasses and squinted to get a good look at him. He still had the cute, crooked smile that I remembered and that bad boy haircut. Because of my skates, I stood a few inches taller than him. He didn't seem as muscular as I had remembered. I couldn't put my finger on it, but something was different.

"You look great," he said. I knew I was sweaty, and my hair was pulled back tightly into an unflattering ponytail, but I had been hoping to hear that.

As the three of us made small talk at a picnic table in the sunshine in front of the Rock and Roll Hall of Fame, it occurred to me what was different. It wasn't Christian's arrogant confidence or his looks that had changed. There wasn't anything different about *him* at all. It was *me*. I had found the strength that I was looking for, and it had changed everything.

Christian never mentioned our last conversation at Green Mountain College. Why would he? I'm sure he didn't even remember. But as I rolled back to the "Big Dog," I let out what felt like the last breath of Christian, no longer desperate to prove myself to him or to anyone. Abandoning Colorado didn't make me a failure. It put me on a bigger path, and I was exactly where I was supposed to be.

On June 16, the day we crossed the Indiana state line, I opened an email from Dad, a difficult man to impress.

Molly,

I am really proud of what you are doing, not just the cause, but also the organization and follow-through. I think you must be about 1/3 of the distance and have covered three of eight states. You're getting there. Please be really careful on the roads. Try not to stop in tight places like we did the other day when I was visiting in Sandusky and the cop made us move.

Love,
Dad

My father wasn't one to show emotion or give too much praise. The only two times I'd ever seen him cry were when his own father died and when I had been in the hospital and my NG tube was harshly removed. But that email, straightforward as it was, said a lot, and on that day, I knew Dad really was proud that I was his daughter.

On our first day in Indiana, a young man saw me out skating against a wall of wind and introduced himself.

I explained about my colon cancer and Rolling to Recovery and jokingly asked if he'd like to keep me company for a while. To my surprise, he drove home, got his bike, and showed up a few miles down the road.

After we parted ways a few hours later, Mom and I pulled the "Big Dog" into the parking lot of a small pizzeria and were discussing that night's dinner when there was a knock at the door and a young woman with a large splotch of marinara on her apron introduced herself.

"What are you doing?" she asked. "What are all the signs?" She pointed at the side of the "Big Dog."

She listened as Mom told the story.

"That's incredible," she said. Then she disappeared.

A few minutes later, Mom and I went in to order some dinner. "I took up a collection!" the woman exclaimed, handing a wad of cash to Mom. "And we have a pizza in the oven for you."

Every day we met people eager to do anything they could to help spread the message that anyone could get colon cancer.

On Friday, June 25, Mom and I rolled into Chicago, our halfway point, for a much needed few days of rest. It was the same day I wore a hole through the inside heel of my right skate, giving me the first blister of the trip. Sergei flew in for the weekend, and we recharged. Brand new skates arrived in an overnight delivery, and when we hit the road again on Monday morning, we began counting the miles down instead of up.

On the outskirts of town, we stopped at a hockey camp to greet a few of the players from the 1998 U.S. women's gold-medal-winning ice hockey team. I didn't tell Mom that I had skipped a final exam in college to watch TV and see them win that medal in Nagano. There was little hope that I would ever play a high level of hockey like that, but I'd found another way to use my passion for skating that was bigger than me, and in a strange way, I was becoming OK with that.

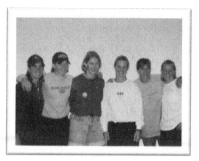

**Collen Coyne, Chris Bailey, Me,
Brandy Fischer, Cammie Granato, Shelley Looney**

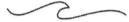

Wednesday, July 5, 2000

Molly,

We're checking your progress almost every day and we are amazed! The boys are learning geography from your trip!! Of course, now they think we can all skate to Colorado! Why drive right?!? Anyway, keep it up, we're all rooting for you!

Love ya,
Cousin Justin, Karen, J.T., Ryan, and David

As the Illinois roads wore on, I had to lean far into the headwind to make any progress. The wind and hills were catching up with me, and my body was growing tired and achy. I was almost ready to give up for the day when I saw a beautiful red-winged blackbird. It took off from its spot on the telephone wire above me and flew a hundred or so feet ahead, before landing back on the wire, where it tipped its head and watched me. I saw a bird like it a few months earlier. My heart surged with emotion.

Back in the spring, while still in the planning stages for Rolling to Recovery, I was walking down the road at Mom and Dad's and remembering Marie, my sweet friend who had lost her battle with colon cancer. As I strolled along, I heard chirping and looked up to see a beautiful, jet black bird with a striking reddish-orange mark on its wing – just like the pin she had given me. It landed on a branch above me and tilted its head, as though saying, "I'm right here." I had walked home with tears in my eyes.

I caught my breath and rolled to a stop in the middle of the road.

"Molly, are you OK?" Mom's voice crackled through the walkie-talkie attached to my CamelBak hydration backpack.

"Yeah, Mom, I'm fine --- just needed to catch my breath for a minute."

"Do you need a break? I've got the A/C on in here."

"No," I said into the walkie-talkie again. "I'm good."

I looked back up at the bird with the reddish-orange mark sitting over me on the wire with its head tilted in the same way I'd observed in the spring. I touched my fingertips to the pin Marie had given me. It was attached to my CamelBak and next to the angel pin Aunt Betty had given me in Chicago. I took a deep breath, smiled, and began striding toward Colorado once more.

The black bird with the orange feathers continued to fly ahead, land, and wait for me to pass her, before doing it all over again. She remained with me as I crossed over the mighty Mississippi the next day, and I caught glances of her throughout the rest of the trip.

15

ROLLING TO RECOVERY
PART TWO

July 10, 2000

Molly,

Read an article about your journey in the radiation oncology waiting room. I'm 23 and have been diagnosed with Hodgkin lymphoma. When I read the story, I felt full of energy and thought it was a very high goal. Today I was so happy to open your page and see you rolling to Colorado. Only young people like you are gonna make CANCER PART OF HISTORY. *My best wishes in all those miles you're gonna roll. I hope this is the first step to make a national roll.* CONGRATULATIONS!!!

You definitely inspire cancer patients and survivors.

Gail

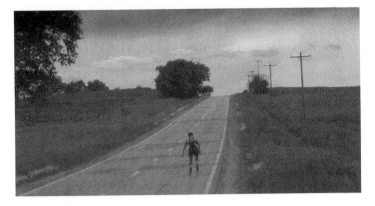

Somewhere in Iowa

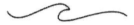

I'd heard that the heat in Iowa and Nebraska in the middle of July could be pretty brutal. That's what I was expecting as I crossed the creaky old toll bridge into Omaha, with Mom right behind me, both of us crossing our fingers that it wouldn't collapse under the weight of our precious "Big Dog." For some reason, I thought the hills would end abruptly on the end of that bridge, but they rolled on – not nearly as tall as the ones that challenged me in New York, but tall enough to make me work.

Outside of Lincoln, Nebraska, we were greeted by Wendell G. Prochaska, the president of the Holiday Rambler RV Club. I hadn't met any long-term survivors of colon cancer until Wendell joined our crusade and happily shared our message through local television and radio shows. I found much hope when he told me he had just celebrated his own 15-year "cancerversary."

Wendell and his wife helped Mom and me survive the streets of Lincoln, where it was illegal to in-line skate. Before we parted ways, he handed me a poem.

A few months ago, or so I've heard,
A plan was put into place.
"Mom, I'd like to skate a while,
but it won't be part of a race."

"I'd like to make my story known
and let myself be heard."
"Even if you're young and strong,
perfect health is not assured."

"My message is pretty simple,
but I hope it will have some clout.
If you hurt for no good reason,
go see a doctor, check it out."

"If I can make a difference,
and make young people hear,
It will be worth the pain and strain,
And yeah, the twinge of fear."

"Trudie will drive the "Big Dog,"
and I'll skate up ahead."
"We'll have the comforts of home,
with a shower, stove and bed."

"Westward Ho!" was Molly's cry
as she headed down the street.
"We'll be in Greeley by late July,
and lots of old friends I'll meet."

New York, Pennsylvania,
"Hey, this ain't bad."
"Kinda rough and hilly,
but cool weather makes me glad."

Ohio, Indiana,
"Wait a minute here."
"Nobody told me there were so many states
between home and way out there."

Illinois, Land of Lincoln,
Chicago, the Windy City,
"I'm going to take a break right now,
my tootsies need lots of pity."

We cross the Mississippi,
We're in the Tall Corn State,
Iowa is the real Midwest,
Hope the rain doesn't make us late.

Wow, it's beastly hot out here,
And Nebraska's really big.
I see lots of horses and cows,
But not one lousy pig.

You say Nebraska's land is flat?
You better think again.
I'll bet the pioneer's horses
Were really, really thin.

The trip is almost over,
Which makes me happy and sad.
Do it again? ... I think not,
But what a time I've had.

The folks I've met, the sights I've seen,
The experience of the road.
I'll remember this trip for the rest of my life,
And I'll know I did lots of good.

Wendell G. Prochaska 7/2000

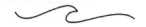

July 13, 2000

Molly, I'm in awe of your willpower, your strength (especially after going through chemo) and your commitment to your cause. I told everyone in the chemo room about you. You made an impression! YOU GO GIRL!

Love,
Nancy

Each morning, I called my radio station back home. I also wrote a weekly column for *The Post-Star,* my local newspaper. New York State's entire North Country was watching from afar and supporting their hometown girl. That's why a call from New York, while we were somewhere in western Nebraska, wasn't surprising.

"Hi, Molly. My name is Pete. I work with the New York Apple Association. I've been following your progress in the newspaper and on the radio. We, the New York Apple Association that is, are one of the sponsors of the New York City Marathon. This year, we've decided that it would be great to enter a cancer survivor to help us get our message out. Cornell University recently published an article about the phytochemicals in apples that help prevent cancer."

"An apple a day, right?" I said.

"Exactly! You already know the catch phrase! We think you would be the perfect spokesperson to run the marathon, tell your story to the media and help us promote the healthy, cancer-fighting qualities of apples."

"*What?*" I was shocked. "I didn't know you could skate in the New York City Marathon."

"I don't think you can. They want you to run!"

I was silent for a moment. "And exactly how far is this marathon?"

"It's 26.2 miles," he said. "You're already in great shape. It shouldn't be a problem."

"Running and skating are two completely different animals," I told him, "and I *hate* running!"

"We'd promote your story too," he said.

"I don't know, Pete."

"We'll put you up in nice hotels and you'll go to New York for interviews."

"Pete, I'd really like to, but I don't think…"

"Molly," he interrupted, "we know you'd be perfect for this."

"But I'm just not a runner. I trip when I walk! You should see me. It's pathetic. That's why I skate instead." I was laughing nervously.

"It's only 26.2 miles," he said. "How far into your journey are you?"

"Probably 1,500 miles, but running is *not* the same."

I liked him, but he just wasn't taking no for an answer. I needed to get off the phone or I knew I would fold.

"Can you give me some time to think about it?"

"Sure," he said. "How about if I give you until Monday?" That was five days --- plenty of time to devise a story about why I *couldn't* run the marathon.

"So, are you going to do it?" Mom asked after I'd hung up.

"Heck no! I don't want to run the New York City Marathon. I don't want to run *any* marathon!"

That afternoon, right on schedule, Rocky called to check my progress.

"How's it going?"

"It's OK. A lot hillier than I thought it was going to be in Nebraska."

"It will get better," he said confidently.

"I got a call this morning from some guy who wants to sponsor me to run the New York City Marathon."

"*What?* The New York City Marathon?" Rocky exclaimed through fits of laughter. "You're not a runner! You told him no way, right?"

"He wouldn't take no for an answer. I told him that I'd would think about it and get back to him."

"Running sucks," he said. "No one should run unless being chased. You can't run 26.2 miles. That's crazy."

"I could if I wanted to," I said.

"I couldn't run 26.2 miles and I doubt you could either."

"I could too," I argued. I couldn't believe Rocky was telling me that I *couldn't* do anything.

"You *can't* run a marathon!" he continued.

"Sure, I can!"

We bickered about the marathon until I got off the phone. I couldn't believe he had the nerve to tell me I couldn't do it.

For the next few days I battled with myself, and I was furious with Rocky. Sure, I hated running, but there was nothing I *couldn't* do.

By the time Pete called back, my mind was made up.

"I really hate running, you know," I reminded him. "My friend Rocky told me that I wouldn't be able to do it."

"So, you won't do it?"

"No," I said. "That's exactly why I'm going to. And I'm going to finish even if I have to crawl!"

As I hung up the phone, I realized I'd been had. Rocky had just pulled the old Jedi mind trick on me. He would never have told me I couldn't do anything unless he wanted me to prove it to him.

July 13, 2000

Molly,

I know you are very busy, but I wanted to check and see how things are going. I think of you often. Hopefully I'll get the chance to talk to you soon! I had a colonoscopy on June 5, and everything is great. It has been a year and four months since my surgery and nine months since I finished chemo, and all is well. I hope the same for you.

Amanda Sherwood

On the road it was at least 90 degrees, but "a dry heat," as everyone liked to tell me. Nightly tornado warnings kept us alert, but as we neared the Colorado border, each morning was more beautiful than the last. It was almost surreal when some of my old hockey teammates drove out to skate with me for a few days, as it signaled that the end of journey was drawing near. I wasn't ready.

We crossed the Colorado border under endless blue sky and got a call from *American Hockey Magazine*. They wanted to meet me in Greeley on my final day to do a story and take the magazine's cover photo. What better way to share the message about colon cancer than in a hockey magazine, where no one is talking about colon cancer.

Molly,

I am still so amazed at what you are accomplishing. (Envious also.) What you are doing is so wonderful. I wish I could do something as courageous.

Anyway, my children are wonderful. Thanks for asking. Caroline, five, is turning into more of a sassy little know-it-all every day, and William, two in September, is starting to look more and more like a little boy. They are both just growing up so fast, and I am so thankful that I'm here to see it. I can't even fathom them having to grow up without me. I think that's what scared me the most about having colon cancer, not that I could die, but that my children wouldn't have their mother. And thanks to people like you who are doing such wonderful things for funding and awareness, I will probably be around for a long time. I hope there are a lot of people who tell you how much you are appreciated.

I hope all is well with you as I am thinking of you and praying that you have a safe and speedy journey.

Please keep in touch and know how special you are.

Amanda

Thirty miles southeast of Greeley, we stopped for a break and let everything sink in. Rocky came out to meet us and the three of us drove to Denver for lunch.

"You should keep skating through the Rockies straight to the West Coast," Rocky joked. He didn't know that that idea had already crossed my mind.

It was strange remembering the last time we had spoken face to face. It had been after his birthday dinner, the night I had gone home and thrown up my chicken Caesar salad, but it felt like we had just been on the ice together the day before.

Hi Molly!

Tomorrow is the big day! Enjoy!
Your parents must be very proud of you and they have every right to be. Godspeed!

> *Love,*
> *Nancy*

I woke on August 31, 2000 and checked the Rolling to Recovery online guestbook.

Molly,

One drop of rain ripples the entire pond. Your life has touched more people than you could have imagined. I still can't say the words 'cancer survivor.' This hasn't been real. Yet, I read your story and found comfort in your strength.

You are not alone. There are many of us.

Thanks for the inspiration. May your life be long, cancer-free and happy.

> *Good luck,*
> *Sean*

I was ready to skate the last miles.

A photographer from *American Hockey Magazine* arrived. Dr. Martelo called to wish me luck, and the owner of the radio stations back home surprised us by arriving in person to live broadcast the big finish.

Nearly 50 old teammates and Colorado friends joined me for the finish with skates, bikes and baby joggers -- my old roommate, Rocky, Holly, Nat, Maddie, Jesse and Eliza.

We hit the road about 10:30 a.m. and made quick work of the final 12 miles. "One mile to go!" a stranger shouted, as he handed me a single red rose. A bittersweet feeling swept through me. Despite all the wind, heat, hills, rain and tornado touchdowns, I wasn't ready for it all to end.

As I turned a corner and headed to JBS Sports Center, I heard a band playing. Everyone fell back, and I crossed the yellow-and-purple paper finish line alone before being swallowed up by friends, cameras and reporters.

"Molly, will you ever put skates on again?" one reporter asked.

I laughed. "I'm playing in a roller hockey game tonight!"

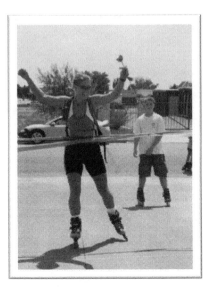

Mel and Jaquie Churchill, Akron News-Reporter

Crossing the Finish Line in Greeley, Colorado

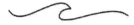

When the champagne had run dry and my friends had disappeared, I could finally start to process what we had just accomplished. We raised over $60,000. For 71 days, Mom and I had lived on top of one another. We had beaten wind, heat, hills and rain. We covered eight states and two thousand miles. I went through three pairs of skates and 100 wheels traveling from Glens Falls, New York to Greeley, Colorado, to get the message out that anyone could get colon cancer, no matter their age. Millions of people saw what the young woman and her mother from the little town in upstate New York were up to, and they started conversations about colon cancer, a disease no one wants to talk about.

Yet I knew my job wasn't complete. I had been given a purpose, and if I could save just one person, it would all be worth it.

September 17, 2000

Hi Molly!

As the subject indicates, I feel like I'm going through withdrawal, since I don't have your diary to read every day. I hope you're enjoying a much-deserved and much needed rest. I'm still "blown away" by what you've done.

I had a CT scan yesterday and will see my doctor tomorrow. My blood work is good, but I just don't trust those blood tests that look for cancer cells. I had one done every three months between my two surgeries and they were always "normal," and yet I had cancer. I have more faith in the scan. I'll be anxious to learn what it shows.

Oh! One more thing. Eric Lindros is leaving the Flyers, as I'm sure you're aware. My son always said you're as good as he is. Why not give it a shot? I'm sure Katie Couric would stand up and take notice then!

Love,
Nancy

On November 5, 2000, three months after I skated across the finish line in Greeley, Sarah and I ran the New York City Marathon together --- or at least for as long as I could keep up with her. At mile 18, I told her to go ahead without me, but once we separated my world crumbled. Everything seemed to hit me at once. I had been diagnosed with colon cancer. I had two major surgeries and then received chemotherapy. I would be under the close care of a doctor for probably the rest of my life. No matter what I wanted, no matter how fast I ran or how hard I skated, I would never escape it. I would forever be a cancer patient.

I limped over the finish line alone, feeling weak and out of control, very much the opposite of my finish three months earlier. The marathon was one of the hardest things I'd ever put my body through *on purpose*. My hips hurt. My knees hurt. The bottoms of my feet hurt. My whole body hurt, but as I soaked in the hotel bathtub that evening, my world came back into focus. Maybe I would be under a doctor's care for the rest of my life, but I had beaten cancer. I was alive, and I had just proven to Rocky and, once again to myself, that I could do anything. I was a strong survivor with a loud voice, and I was nowhere near finished showing the world.

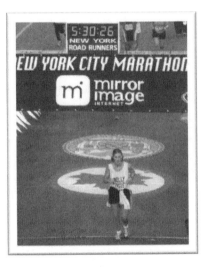

Finishing the New York City Marathon

16

SOMEONE LIKE ME

The year 2000, *my* year, rolled into 2001, and things began to settle down. Because I enjoyed being on the radio so much during my trip, I accepted an offer to become an on-air personality at Cool Rock 95.9 FM, one of the local stations that had followed my journey. I was back at home, enjoying family and spending time with Sergei.

I continued my email friendships with Amanda and Nancy. Because we were about the same age, Amanda and I were becoming especially close. We didn't always talk about cancer. We shared our everyday lives and slowly learned about each other as friends, not perpetual patients. I couldn't believe that Amanda and I went through practically the same things at almost the same time, but we lived 1,000 miles away from each other.

One day, we had a light-hearted chat via instant message.

Amanda: You and Sergei should meet me and my Dad in North Carolina. I found a place to swim with the dolphins. I've always wanted to do that. We could meet!

Molly: That sounds awesome and I have to admit that it would be fun to wander down the beach together in bikinis, scaring all of the little children with our matching scars.

Amanda: You're too funny.

Molly: Amanda, how were you actually diagnosed?

Amanda: I was pregnant with my second child when I first started having symptoms.

Molly: What kind of symptoms?

Amanda: Rectal bleeding, throwing up and I had some abdominal pain.

Molly: Same as me.

Amanda: My doctors told me that it was the pregnancy, but I knew something wasn't right. I'd been pregnant before and it just didn't feel the same, but they insisted. I had a C-Section in September of 1998, but by Thanksgiving, when the pain was still there, I went back to my doctor. He told me it was probably just an ulcer and blamed it on stress.

Molly: Wow!

Amanda: In early December, I called him again and told him that there was blood in my stool. That's when he ordered stool cultures and tested for parasites and eggs. The week before Christmas, his nurse called and told me that the tests were negative --- no parasites.

Amanda: When I told the nurse that I was still having symptoms, she said to "just wait and they will probably go away."

Molly: Unbelievable! But somehow not surprising.

Amanda: Sometime in January, I remember going to the bathroom -- you know, number two --- and when I wiped, it was like I had started my period, but it was coming from the wrong place. I went to see my doctor the next day.

Amanda: He read my chart and found that the same nurse who had told me to "just wait" had missed an order to send me in for a colonoscopy if the original test came back negative.

Molly: Same stupid story! Misdiagnosed because you're too young to have cancer!

Amanda: My insurance company thought it was ridiculous that I would need a colonoscopy too.

Molly: But you got one, right?

Amanda: My doctor fought with them to get it.

Molly: Did they agree to pay for it?

Amanda: Of course not. The doctor was ready to pay for it out of his own pocket and went ahead with it anyway. In the end, since I had cancer, the insurance company paid without a fight. On January 26, 1999, I was diagnosed with Stage III metastatic adenocarcinoma. I was 24.

Molly: Don't you love those big words? Why don't they just say it like it is – stupid colon cancer?

Amanda: No kidding! Then it was on to chemo. I started in March of 1999, with 5-FU and leucovorin.

Molly: That's what I did. Four cycles? Four weeks on and two off?

Amanda: That's what I started with, but I had a really bad reaction. Threw up and had diarrhea for a week. Then I had to be treated in the emergency room before they finally lowered my dosage.

I didn't want to tell Amanda that while she was having a negative reaction to the chemo, I continued to play hockey once a week and in-line skated to my treatments when I felt up to it. How could we have had such different reactions to the same chemo?

Amanda: As if life weren't bad enough, my husband couldn't handle it and that's when we decided to separate.

Molly: Amanda, I'm so sorry. How long were you together?

Amanda: Just under three years, but it's OK. At least I found out early on in our marriage. And I have two beautiful children.

Molly: Did the doctors keep you on the 5-FU and leucovorin?

Amanda: Yup, and I finished on September 27, 1999.

Molly: One month before me!

Amanda: The timeline is so similar.

Molly: Almost scary. How often do you have checkups now?

Amanda: Every few months. I had my first checkup in January of 2000 and everything was good – for a while, anyway. The doctors told me that because I was diagnosed in Stage III, there was a great possibility that my cancer would return, but for the time, I was just happy to be alive and enjoying my children.

Molly: Then what happened?

Amanda: In August of 2000, it came back in my abdomen. I started doing treatments again, but the doctors told me they were no longer working and that my tumor was inoperable. That's when I stopped chemo.

In August of 2000, I had just finished Rolling to Recovery and was training for the 2000 New York City Marathon. Why did her cancer come back?

Amanda: So, I'm fighting again! Even though things don't look so good for me, I'm not going to let it get me down. I will fight this battle to the end!

Molly: And I'll be right here with you!

After Amanda told me her story, I kept asking myself why I was the one who had beaten it and she still had to fight. I knew about survivor's guilt but never understood it until I became friends with someone so young who was still fighting a beast that was easy to beat if it was caught early enough.

As Amanda's fight wore on, she tried different drugs and clinical trials, and her personal emails became group emails.

July 14, 2001

Hello to all of you!

All of our prayers are working. We got good news in Houston! I was very surprised and very excited. I was expecting the worst. Every time I go down there, I have a blood test called a CEA. This is normal when it is 3 or below. A CEA count above 3 is bad. In March my CEA was 3. On June 1, my CEA was 30. On Friday, my CEA was down to 18!!!!! Still high, but lower. This is a sign that my new chemo is having an effect on my tumor. Also, last time I had fluid around my lungs, and I did not have full function of my lungs. Apparently, the fluid is gone, and I have full function of my lungs back. The only things my doctors were unhappy with were my weight loss (15 pounds in a month) and that my red cell count is low, which they have tried to remedy with a shot of Procrit. They seemed very pleased and even kind of surprised at how well I'm doing after just two weeks on chemo. I know that God is taking care of me and answering all our prayers. Thank you all so much. Things are so difficult in my life right now and it means so much to know that I have so many prayers being said for me.

Love you!
Amanda

As I read her words, relief poured through me. Someday, we would prance around on a beach together, sporting bikinis and scars. Were there others like us out there? Had any of them found each other the way we had?

July 23, 2001

Hey guys!

I just wanted to say hi to everyone and let you all know what's going on with me. As you know, I started my new chemo (seven pills a day) on June 25. The chemo is actually one of the common treatments for breast cancer and pretty recently has been used on colon cancer. It is called Xeloda ("zee-lo-da"). The side effects are very mild, especially since I take it every single day for 14 days straight. So far, I'm handling it really well. I guess my eating habits aren't so great, but they are getting better. I haven't been physically sick once (although I've come close a couple of times). I wouldn't say I feel great, but good. I tire easily and I'm sure that is a combination of the cancer and the chemo. The only problem I'm having is one of the side effects is Hand-Foot Syndrome, and the bottoms of my feet are very sensitive. Summer is going great! I've taken the kids swimming some, and it's been nice spending time with them.

Love,
Manda

Amanda's group emails continued to arrive, but then they became less and less frequent. I shrugged it off, thinking she was busy because she was feeling better. I wrote back whenever I heard from her or if I had a funny story to share. I was concentrating on moving on with my life. Then one evening I got a call that would forever change my path.

"Hello. Could I please speak with Molly McMaster?" The voice sounded like a woman about my age.

"This is Molly," I answered.

"I'm doing PR for Chevrolet, and the Olympic Torch Relay. Have you heard about us?" she asked.

"Um, yes, I think so," I said. One of my teammates on my women's hockey team had asked if she could nominate me to carry the Olympic Torch. A co-worker at the radio station also said they nominated me, but I hadn't thought much of it. I was excited just to be considered.

"Chevrolet has been running a promotion where people can nominate someone that they believe is inspiring to carry the Olympic Torch, and you have been chosen as one of our inspirational Torchbearers."

"What?"

"I'm calling to let you know that you've been selected to carry the 2002 Olympic Torch on its way to Salt Lake City, Utah."

"*What?*" I repeated, standing up from my seat on the couch. "You're kidding!" A chill went up my spine.

"A woman in Little Rock, Arkansas nominated you," she continued. "Do you know a young woman by the name of Amanda Sherwood-Roberts?"

I fell silent and ghost white. I felt like I had a lump in my throat, and I couldn't speak.

"Molly? Do you know her?" she asked again.

I was on the verge of tears, both of joy and sadness.

"Yes, I know her," I finally forced out.

"Molly, what she wrote about you was so touching. You're a colon cancer survivor? Diagnosed at 23? Is that right?"

"You don't understand," I interrupted. "Amanda is my age and *also* has colon cancer. We're the only two in the country this young that either of us knows about. We've never met in person."

The next day I found Amanda's home phone number in an old email. I had never spoken on the phone with her, but I wanted to thank her.

"Hello?" A man with a Southern drawl answered the phone.

"Hi," I said timidly. "I'm trying to reach Amanda. This is her friend Molly from New York."

"Molly? How are ya? This is Bernie, Amanda's Dad! We've heard so much about ya!" I couldn't believe it. Amanda had been talking to her family about me the same way that I talked about her. "'Manda will be so happy to hear from ya! 'Manda!" he shouted. My hand was shaking as I held the phone. I hoped it was OK that I called.

"Hello?" It was so nice to finally put a voice with the pictures that she had sent me.

"Amanda?" I said. "It's Molly."

"Hi," she said in her polite Southern drawl. "How are you?" She sounded like she had been expecting to hear from me, but she was weak, and I finally grasped how sick she was and why her emails were so infrequent. She wasn't busy playing with her children. She was busy fighting stupid cancer. I felt ashamed calling to tell her my exciting news while she was battling for her life.

"I'm good," I said. "How are you?"

"I'm OK," she said. "Started a new treatment a few weeks ago, and it doesn't agree too well with me, but I'm hanging in there."

"How are your kids?" I asked, trying to dodge the real reason that I had called.

"They're good. Causing trouble, as usual," she giggled.

"Isn't that what kids are supposed to do?" I laughed with her through my nervousness. "Amanda, I got some really incredible news yesterday that I wanted to share with you. Someone I know in Little Rock, Arkansas nominated me to carry the Olympic Torch, and apparently I've been chosen."

"Really?" she said.

"Yeah. Can you believe it?"

"Molly, that's so great. Congratulations!" She was excited and proud for both of us, but her voice changed only slightly as she spoke, as if she was trying to speak louder. I knew the cancer was to blame. "I wish I could be doing those things with you. But you're going to have to do them until I get better and can join you."

"You got it." I said.

I hung up the phone and let Amanda's battle really sink in. The mood of her emails was always light, sweetened so our concern would be minimal. In most of them, Amanda seemed matter-of-fact and not worried. But after speaking to her, I understood how weak and sick she really was. She had nominated me to carry the torch, to fight back against a disease that was beating her. I couldn't let her down.

August 27, 2001

Hey guys!

We just got back in from Houston. As I expected, my appointment didn't go well. My chemotherapy is not working, and my tumor is continuing to grow. It was at 11 cm in May, and it is at 15 cm right now.

My CEA count went up from 18 to 36, which is the highest it has ever been. Other than that, my blood counts are great, and my weight has stayed exactly the same!

On a brighter note, I leave for Hawaii in one week and six days!!!!! I am very excited! I had an awful dream that I missed my flight. Wouldn't that be the worst thing?!

As soon as I hear from the doctor, I will let you all know what is going on. Like I said, feel free to email or call with any questions. Again, thank you all for your constant support and prayers. It means so much to my family and me to have such wonderful people in our lives!

Love you all!
Amanda

17

LITTLE ROCK

The second week of September, I got a call from *The Early Show* on CBS. They heard my story through the PR company for the Chevy Olympic Torch Bearers and wanted me to do an interview with Bryant Gumbel. I emailed all my friends, telling them about the interview, which was scheduled on September 12, 2001.

Molly,

I'll be in New York City that day too! Could I please take you out for lunch at Tavern on the Green? It's really a beautiful restaurant, and I'd love to meet you and take you there.

Love,
Nancy

It would be wonderful. I would talk about colon cancer on national television and meet my other email buddy, all in the same day. I was so excited.

On September 11, 2001, I woke up early, packed, and did my morning workout while watching Bryant Gumbel on TV. I was ticketed on a train to New York City that afternoon and was still debating which outfit to wear for the interview the following morning. As I ran on the treadmill and thought about the questions Gumbel might ask, two planes struck two buildings in New York City.

I didn't board the train that afternoon and I didn't meet Nancy. Instead, I sat in front of the television, terrified for myself, my friends, my family and my country. Colon cancer was the last thing on my mind.

A few weeks later, when the shock began to wear off, I questioned my campaign. How important was it for me to teach people about colon cancer when terrorists were hijacking airplanes and flying them into buildings in our country, killing thousands of people?

Then, one Monday night in early November, I found an email in my inbox from a stranger.

Dear Molly,

You don't know me, but my name is Hannah and I am Amanda's cousin (well, one of many!). She doesn't know that I am emailing you. I found your website on the Internet. I know the two of you have never met in person, but I also know that Amanda was really hoping that she would get the chance someday. We have talked about her coming to NYC (where I live) and somehow getting together with you. She has told me that you are the only person who really understands what she has gone through because there aren't that many young women diagnosed with colon cancer.

I don't know if Amanda has written you lately, but she is doing badly. She is at home and has started hospice care (right now, just morphine and other drugs). I don't know how you would feel about this, but some of us in the family were hoping that you might consider letting us get you a plane ticket to Little Rock so that Amanda can meet you. She is having a birthday party on November 23 (her 27th, the day after Thanksgiving) and I would love for you to be there, but it might be better to come as soon as possible.

Sorry to ambush you with this in an email. I don't know if you would feel comfortable doing this or not and I would completely understand if you didn't want to. If you wouldn't mind me calling you, please write me back with your phone number and a good time to call.

I hope all continues to be well with you.

Take care,
Hannah

When I finished reading the letter, my heart was pounding and tears were spilling down both cheeks. I was elated with the idea of meeting Amanda, but part of me was terrified. I wanted to believe that she was getting her life back. Instead, at age 26, it was being taken away. As I read the email again, I felt a calm come over me. I saw clearly why I was fighting. Terrorists were attacking. War was looming on the horizon, but people were still dying of colon cancer here in our own country.

I would go to Little Rock, and I would go that weekend. "Definitely! Call me tomorrow," I typed, "sometime after six!" I hit the reply button and glanced at the clock. There was so much I wanted to say to Hannah, but I had to be on the ice for hockey practice in 45 minutes.

The next day, I sent a mass email to everyone I knew. I would go to Little Rock, but I didn't want Amanda's family to pay for it.

By the time Hannah and I connected, a frequent flier ticket had been given to me by a friend of a friend, and I planned to go to Little Rock as soon as possible. I loved Hannah from minute one. She was spunky, friendly and outgoing.

That Friday, I headed to the airport to meet Benita Zahn, a reporter from WNYT, the NBC affiliate in Albany, New York. Benita had covered much of my story so far, from skating across the country and running the New York City Marathon to speaking to local schools and community groups about colon cancer. But she seemed most taken with my trip to Little Rock to meet Amanda, the "other girl" with colon cancer.

"Molly, are you bringing anything special for Amanda?" she asked, smiling at the camera. I pulled a few small stuffed animals from my bag.

"These are for Caroline and William, her two kids," I said. "And this is for her." I held my hand open for the camera to show a piece of metal no bigger than a quarter.

"And what's that?" she asked.

"It's a pocket angel," I said. "While I was doing chemotherapy in 1999, I was the assistant coach of the Nineteen and Under Adirondack Northstars Girls Ice Hockey Team out of Glens Falls. One evening at practice, one of the girls handed it to me. She and her mother wanted me to have an angel to watch over me. It worked for me. I'm hoping it can give Amanda a miracle as well." As I said the words, I realized that I was fiddling with my pewter necklace, the one that Sarah gave me. I always wore it when I was scared or nervous. I wore it through chemo. I wore it at the Empire State Games, every day during

Rolling to Recovery and in the New York City Marathon. It was around my neck during all of my follow-up medical tests, X-rays and CT Scans. Now I was wearing it on my visit to Amanda in Arkansas.

When I arrived in Little Rock a few hours later, Hannah and some of her family met me at the airport. "Trust me. There are a lot more of us," she said. After a few hugs and a phone call to be sure that Amanda was awake, we piled into the car and left the airport.

I was nervous when I walked into the house, but Amanda's father quickly put me at ease. "Molly, our house is your house," Bernie said.

"You sure you want to tell me that?" I joked.

"Queenie? You awake?" he shouted down the hallway in the direction of what I assumed was Amanda's bedroom. "She's the queen of the house, so I call her Queenie." He laughed and winked at me. We waited for a few moments and didn't hear a reply. "Queenie?" he shouted again. "Molly's here!"

"I'm comin', dang it!" Amanda's feisty voice from down the hall sounded much better than when I had talked to her on the phone. Maybe she really was getting better. Maybe they were all wrong about her cancer and I was the only one who could tell. But when she stepped into the light of the living room, I saw the emaciated frame of a very beautiful and very sick girl. I felt ashamed that I was in such good health. Did she hate me for surviving the monster? Maybe this trip hadn't been such a great idea.

"It's about time you got here, girl," she said, easing my awkwardness, and I laughed as I walked toward her.

"Those darned pilots are always taking their sweet time," I said, reaching gently around her, afraid that if I hugged her too tightly she might break. It was shocking to see only a shell of the girl who had emailed me her picture just a few months before. I wanted to cry as I looked into her dark and sunken eyes and held her fragile hands. I could see that she was in discomfort. Why was this happening to her? And why didn't it happen to me?

After hugs from Amanda, Bernie and Amanda's mom, Martha, we sat in the living room and chatted. Amanda was lying on a couch with a hot water bottle on her belly and her feet in her mother's lap. The light dose of morphine made her drowsy. Her eyes were closed but she wasn't sleeping. She listened, and when she heard something of interest, she piped up to chat and joke.

I watched her for a few minutes, finding it strange that everyone was talking about everyday things and ignoring the tumor in her belly. Maybe not talking about it helped them think it wasn't happening.

"I spoke to my friend Sarah during my layover," I said. "She couldn't believe I was going to visit a bunch of people I had never met before. 'You're going to Little Rock alone? What if they're mass murderers?' she asked. I had to admit that for a moment, I did get a little bit nervous." We all laughed, except Amanda.

"Mom?" she asked.

"Yes, Amanda?"

"Could you get me the phone?"

"What for? It's almost midnight."

"I want to call Sarah and demand $50,000 or she'll never see her friend again and we'll bury her in the backyard." We all burst into laughter. I was amazed. Through all the pain, somehow Amanda kept her sense of humor.

We stayed up late into the night talking about our families, the weather and the tornado that had swept through their neighborhood a few years earlier. But no one talked about the cancer --- not mine, and not Amanda's.

On Saturday morning, a local news crew was scheduled to arrive. I put on minimal makeup, not wanting Amanda to appear sickly in comparison, and sat with her as she flawlessly applied her own makeup. Before we left her room, I pulled the coin-shaped angel from my pocket.

"Amanda, I have something for you," I said, holding out my hand.

"What's this?" she asked, gently picking it up.

"It's a pocket angel. It's supposed to watch over you," I said.

"Molly, thank you so much," Amanda said, smiling as she put it into her pocket.

With Amanda's family watching, we sat together on the couch, holding hands as we answered questions in front of the television camera.

After the news crew left, Amanda took a nap while I watched the home video of her trip to Hawaii, where her dream to swim with dolphins came true. It was only six weeks ago. How could that be? Amanda could barely walk down the hallway now, but on the screen she was running up and down a beach, dancing and swimming with dolphins. Suddenly, I regretted not having our rendezvous at the beach with our bikinis and matching scars, but I couldn't do anything about it now. She had terminal colon cancer. There was no going back.

When Amanda woke up, we went back to sitting on the couch and visiting.

"So, are we gonna compare scars or what?" I asked.

"Heck, yeah," she said. "Let me see yours first!"

"Alright, Alright." I stood and untucked my shirt, pulling it halfway up my rib cage and holding it up to expose my bare belly. "Now, let me see yours!"

Amanda didn't stand up. She handed her Mom the hot water bottle that rested on her belly, then pulled her shirt up the same way that I had.

Our scars were basically the same: vertical lines running down our abdomens for about 10 inches, from the middle of the rib cage to just above the pubic bone. But Amanda's scar was a little different. While my scar passed right next to my belly button, her scar made a crescent-shaped detour, bypassing her belly button.

"What the heck? I may have to sue," she joked. And we both laughed.

That night, when Amanda and I were getting ready to watch *Saturday Night Live* in her room, she started feeling sick. "Amanda, are you OK?" I asked. I grabbed a wastebasket and held it in front of her as she vomited. It felt like I was watching myself just a few years ago. Why didn't I realize then that something serious was wrong with me? Why hadn't I pushed my doctor? Why didn't Amanda push her doctor for an answer?

I wanted to help her but knew there was nothing I could do. Amanda had just drunk some juice with her morphine and that damned tumor wouldn't let anything through. I rubbed her back, held the bucket, and wished that she would get better.

When the vomiting ended, we cleaned up and watched most of *Saturday Night Live*. It was our first time alone together, but we didn't talk much. We didn't have to. We were like old friends, sharing a bond understood only by us. She laid in bed with her feet in my lap. Everyone told me that she loved to have her feet rubbed. That's exactly what I did.

"Molly, I have to admit that I'm jealous of all of the things that you have been doing to raise awareness of colon cancer," she said in the darkness. "I hope you know that if I weren't so sick, I would be right there with you."

I paused before answering. I didn't know how to respond. "I know you would," I said. "I guess I'll just have to keep doing it for both of us."

"Promise?" she asked.

"Promise," I said.

On Sunday morning, I played with Amanda's six-year-old daughter before Amanda got up.

"I brought nail polish!" I told Caroline.

"Really? What colors did you bring?"

"Blue, Red, Purple, Pink. All different colors. I must have at least eight different bottles with me," I said.

"Can we do my nails all different colors?" she begged.

"Absolutely," I said. "You're a girl after my own heart!"

We sat on the kitchen floor, newspaper spread all around us, and I painted Caroline's fingers and toes in every color polish I had. She giggled and told me about what would happen if she wore nail polish to her private Catholic school.

"Just like her mother," Martha said. "Amanda used to get in trouble all the time doing those kinds of things."

I painted the last of Caroline's little piggies, knowing she would probably never have that experience again with her mother. I remembered Amanda telling me that she wasn't scared of dying. She was scared that her children wouldn't have a Mom.

When it was time for me to leave, Amanda's family gave me a t-shirt and blanket emblazoned with an Arkansas Razorback. I also unwrapped a glass angel with hands that were pressed together in prayer. Behind the angel, on a mirror, these words were etched: "The spirit with which you live your life inspires those around you." I forced myself not to cry and hugged Amanda. "I love you," I whispered in her ear. "Keep smiling, I'll be back."

All the doubts I had about going to Arkansas were gone. My only regret was that I had not met Amanda sooner. And somewhere deep down, I found it hard to believe that there wasn't still a way to save her.

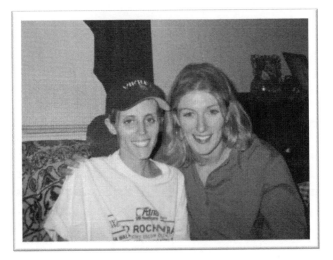

Amanda and Me

18

KATIE

Later that week, I boarded a train to New York City's Penn Station, wishing Amanda were by my side. She adored *Today* show co-host Katie Couric, but her illness would not allow her to travel. Instead, she would do her *Today* interview from her couch in Little Rock, live via satellite. It was so unfair. I was thrilled that we were getting the chance to tell our stories to millions of people who would be watching the show on national TV, but looking even more forward to breaking the stereotype associated with colon cancer. Together, our young faces would prove that it wasn't just a disease that happened to 50-year-old white men. But why did one of us have to be dying for the story to be worth airing in front of an audience?

In the morning, a limo whisked me off to Rockefeller Plaza, home of NBC studios. In the greenroom, where guests waiting for their turn to be interviewed, at least 15 people were stuffed together on two couches.

After 30 minutes, an NBC page stepped into the greenroom.

"Molly, would you like to have your makeup done?"

"Yes, please," I said, feeling like a princess. I followed her down the hall into a room with large mirrors and hair salon chairs. The makeup artist turned me into a movie star. Amanda would have loved it.

Back in the greenroom, I was glamorous and hungry but refused to eat anything lest I smudge my makeup. Instead, I stepped outside of the room and called Amanda one last time before our interview.

"How are you feeling, Amanda?"

"I just threw up, but I'm feeling much better now!" she laughed.

"Was it nerves or are you sick this morning?"

"Just not feeling well," she admitted. "But I'll be fine. I didn't take my full dose of morphine this morning, and I'm sure that's not helping. I want people to be able to understand what I'm saying. I can get pretty out of it when I'm on that stuff. How is it there?"

"It's cool," I said. "I just got back in from makeup. Go heavy on the eyes," I instructed.

While I was talking to Amanda, I noticed that *Today* co-host Matt Lauer was walking toward me from down the hall. He was much shorter than I had imagined he would be.

"I'm sorry," I said to him. "Am I in the way out here?"

"Oh, don't be silly. You're fine," he said. Then he disappeared into the little kitchen across the hall from the greenroom.

"Who was that?" Amanda asked. I felt bad telling her who interrupted our chat. I wanted her to be here with me.

"Um, it was Matt Lauer," I said quietly.

"You jerk!" she said with a giggle.

A few minutes later, I followed another NBC page down a flight of stairs and into a brightly lit studio. I was directed to a chair, connected to a microphone and earpiece and then left alone. I was calm and cool as I surveyed the studio with what looked like thousands of lights on the ceiling and different sets in each corner. Then I glanced toward the front window. When I saw the huge crowd peering in, my heart beat loudly in my ears. I couldn't hear anything else. "Oh, man," I thought. "This is *live.*"

At that same moment, a familiar body with a huge smile appeared in the chair next to me.

"Hi, Molly. I'm Katie Couric," she said. I had to laugh. How ridiculous was it for *her* to be introducing herself to *me?* Wasn't it supposed to be the other way around?

"Hi," I said shyly, keeping my eyes on the crowd outside.

Then Amanda's beautiful face appeared in black-and-white on the screen in front of me. She looked very composed, and her smile calmed me. We were together again to tell our stories, but this time it would be broadcast across the country.

A man stepped in front of us and counted down with his hand. Three fingers. Two. One. He pointed at Katie and she began to speak.

"Three weeks from now, the Olympic Flame will begin to make its way from Atlanta, Georgia to Salt Lake

City, Utah," Katie began. "Among this year's torchbearers is Molly McMaster, who at 25 is a colon cancer survivor. Molly was nominated by a friend she met on the Internet two years ago, Amanda Sherwood Roberts, who at 26 also suffers from the disease. Last weekend, the young women met for the first time. Molly McMaster is here with us this morning, and Amanda Sherwood Roberts is at her home in Arkansas. Good morning to both of you. I'm so happy to see you both."

"Good morning, Katie," I said.

"Good morning," Amanda said sweetly.

"Let me start with you first, Molly. I know that it's quite unusual for someone in their twenties to be diagnosed with colon cancer. You were looking for someone to talk with about your experience on the Internet, and you all met in a chat room. Is that correct?"

"Actually," I began, "Amanda received an email about the *crazy* things I was doing through the Colon Cancer Alliance."

"Tell everyone about what you were doing," Katie laughed.

"Last summer, I in-line skated from Glens Falls, New York, my hometown, to Greeley, Colorado, to raise money and awareness. Then I ran the New York City Marathon. I want to bring awareness about the disease. Crazy things, that's the way to do it."

"Even though it's unusual, young people *are* diagnosed with this disease, but the emphasis is on people 50 and older," Katie said.

"Absolutely," I said. "You need to know your body, know the symptoms and know what they mean. You need to understand and know your body because doctors may not think about cancer in a younger patient."

"Now, Amanda," Katie continued, turning to the black-and-white screen, "Why did you want to reach out to Molly?"

"After doing so much research on the Internet, and looking at information everywhere, she was actually the first person I found that was my age. It was nice to have somebody that could actually relate to my experience. We did find out that we have a whole lot in common," Amanda said.

"You decided that Molly would be the perfect person to be an Olympic Torchbearer, so you actually wrote an essay nominating her, is that right?" Katie asked.

"Yes, Ma'am," Amanda said politely. "She did these crazy things, and I just had so much admiration for her courage to get out there and do that, and just to have so much determination to bring awareness to people who may not know anything about the disease."

"When you found out that Amanda had done this, and that you were in fact, chosen to be a torchbearer, what was your reaction, Molly?" Katie asked me.

"I cried. And when I found out it was Amanda who nominated me, I could *not* believe it. Now it means so much more than it ever could have."

Katie turned toward Amanda on the screen.

"Amanda, what was it like to be able to meet Molly face to face?"

"Oh, it was amazing – absolutely amazing," she said. "That's one thing I really wanted to be able to do, was to be able to meet Molly, and thanks to my cousin, it happened."

"You know, Amanda, it breaks my heart to say that you do have stage IV colon cancer. You also have two children. Caroline is six and William is three?"

"Yes."

"Where do you find the strength to go on national television and talk about this disease?"

"I have a wonderful, wonderful family support network. Without my parents, I think there's a lot that I wouldn't be able to do."

"Amanda, what is the most important thing you'd like people to know about this disease?"

"First of all, listen to your body, especially at mine and Molly's age, because I know I had a lot of trouble trying to get diagnosed, with my insurance company. Be persistent, and when you do get older, get tested. When you've got the family history, get tested, because as we all know colon cancer is one of the most treatable diseases, if you can catch it early."

"That's right," Katie said. "And even if you don't have a family history, it's very important to be screened, because 85 percent of all cases involve no family history at all."

"Amanda Sherwood Roberts, I think you're a very brave and beautiful young woman, and I so appreciate your talking with us. Thank you, Amanda."

"Thank you, Katie," Amanda said.

"Molly McMaster, I wish you lots of luck in the future. You're enjoying good health. I'm very happy to see that, and good luck carrying the torch."

"Thank you, Katie."

"This is a very emotional story for me," Katie said, choking back tears. "We'll be right back."

The interview was five minutes long, but it felt like a mere heartbeat. As the show cut to a commercial, I looked at Katie, who was shaken and wiping away tears. I knew that her husband had died of colon cancer in 1998, when he was only 42 years old, and that her sister had recently lost her battle with another form of cancer. In

2000, Katie underwent a colonoscopy on the *Today* show to raise awareness of colon cancer herself. I wanted to reach over and hug her. I wanted to tell her that this was exactly what Amanda had wanted. She wanted to tell the world how easy it was to *not* get colon cancer, and Katie had given her that opportunity. But instead, I sat and smiled, too nervous to do anything.

"Molly, could you stick around for a little while?" Katie asked me as a makeup artist hid her tears.

"I can," I said.

"I'll meet you in the greenroom when the show's over," she said. "I'd like to speak with you some more."

"Molly, you guys were fantastic," Hannah said when I returned to the greenroom. "The whole room was silent, and by the end, almost everyone in the room was crying. People really listened to the two of you, and I don't think they are going to forget."

"Thanks," I said, somewhat embarrassed. "Katie asked me to wait here until after the show. She's going to come and talk to us."

"Really? That's great!" Hannah said.

When Katie finally appeared, I was somewhat taken aback. She was extremely easygoing and *normal,* not what I expected a celebrity to be. I liked her immensely. Hannah and I kept her ears busy, answering her questions about Amanda and her family. When the tape delay had passed, and we were certain that the piece had aired in Little Rock, Hannah called Amanda on her cell phone.

"Amanda, Katie is standing with us," Hannah said. "Couric, Crazy! Who did you think I meant? She'd like to know if it would be OK to speak with you." We all laughed as Katie took Hannah's phone and walked away to speak privately with Amanda.

When the 30-minute whirlwind was over, Katie signed a few autographs and got a goodie bag together for Amanda. "I hate to do this," she said, "but I'm late for a meeting. Molly, thank you so much for sharing your story." She turned and began to walk toward the door, then turned back to face me. "If you think of anything crazy for Colorectal Cancer Awareness Month in March, let me know. We'll have you back on the show!"

"You got it!" I said.

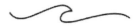

Dear Molly,

You're in the wrong business. You don't belong on the radio. You belong on TV! You're beautiful! The fact that Katie was moved to tears moved me to tears.

I felt like I had met you at last.

Love,
Nancy

19

AN OLYMPIC MOMENT

Two weeks later, I flew to Little Rock again, this time to celebrate Amanda's 27ᵗʰ birthday. When I arrived, I was shocked. The birthday party, the one she had been planning for almost six months, was less than an hour away but she was still in bed.

"Queenie," Bernie whispered into her ear. "You awake? Molly's here."

Amanda opened one eye and then the other.

"Hi, Amanda," I said. "I told you I'd be back."

"Hi," she said softly. Then she sat up and started vomiting. Bernie had the wastebasket at the ready and held it under her mouth.

"I'm better," Amanda said slowly, wiping her mouth with the cloth she kept next to her bed. She sat up and gave me a hug. It was only two weeks ago when I last saw her, but somehow she looked more tired, more undernourished and in more pain.

"How are you doing?" I asked, knowing it was a stupid question but not able to think of anything else to say.

"I'm tired," she admitted. "Need to start getting ready for the party though." Her speech was slow and forced and it was obvious how awful she felt but it was her birthday. No matter how sick she was, the party was going to happen. At first, I found it hard to believe, but remembered my own experience. In the hospital, I was a social butterfly, with so many visitors the nurses had to tell people to go away.

"Molly, you need your rest and you won't sleep when people are here," the nurses scolded.

"But I don't want to miss anything," I had whined.

I smiled, thinking of how similar Amanda and I were. Why couldn't we have had something else in common though? Why couldn't we have met playing hockey or through school? Instead, colon cancer was our commonality. It just wasn't fair.

"What are you going to wear tonight?" I asked her. "I'll help you."

"Pink satin pajamas. They're hanging in my closet. And the pink fuzzy slippers."

When her pajamas and slippers were on, she reached for her brush and makeup bag. She applied her makeup perfectly once again. "Can't forget my tiara," she laughed, sliding it into place on top of her head.

Within the hour, guests began to arrive, and soon the house was full. Amanda lay quietly on the couch, greeting friends and family. As more and more people arrived, they had to line up to talk with her.

I watched from across the room as she threw up. Everyone took the cue and backed away while her parents held her and her wastebasket. When she finished vomiting and slowly wiped her face, people lined up again. It was strange scene.

Late into the evening a few girls showed up and sat with Amanda on the couch, giggling and laughing.

"Who are they?" I asked Hannah.

"Old friends from high school," she said, sounding rather disgusted. "I don't think Amanda has spoken to them since graduation."

"What are they doing here?" I asked.

"Not sure. I heard someone say that someone ran into them at the mall this afternoon and told them about Amanda's party." She looked at me and then shifted her eyes back to Amanda on the couch. "They're probably just here to get a good look." I shook my head. "They probably feel guilty that they haven't spoken to her in so long and now she's dying."

Had people looked at me that way? I remembered getting a phone call from someone I had played hockey with in Colorado. "Molly, are you OK?" he had asked. "I heard that you have cancer and that you're going to *die*," he said. After we spoke that day, I never heard from him again.

I watched Amanda and the four women, who were acting as though Amanda only had a cold.

No one in the room had any idea what Amanda was going through. For a while, I knew, but now Amanda was on her own, venturing into a world that none of us knew or understood.

"Have you come up with anything crazy for Katie yet?" Hannah asked, trying to forget the women with Amanda.

"Oh," I laughed. "No, not yet, but I've been thinking about it."

"My stepmom and I think that you should ride around the country on a zebra," she said.

I laughed again. "OK. I'll bite. You want to explain that one?"

"My stepmom wrote a paper for her nursing students about how when doctors hear hoofbeats, they tend to look for a horse. Sometimes they should be looking for a zebra instead."

"What?" I was lost.

"You and Amanda are the zebras," she continued.

"I got it. I can do that. You know I already ride horses, don't you?"

Hannah and I questioned guests at the party about their knowledge of zebras. Where would we find one? Were they endangered? Could you ride them?

"Zebras bite," someone finally said, stopping our plan cold.

"It was a clever idea," I laughed. "Let's try for something else."

When it was time to leave Little Rock again, it was much more difficult than the first visit. Amanda and I knew that we would probably never see each other again, but those weren't the words we shared.

"I'll see you again soon," I said, giving her a hug and an extra squeeze. I knew now that she was tough and wouldn't break. "I love you."

"I love you too," she whispered.

I left the house smiling. I hated what was happening, but because of cancer, I had the opportunity to know Amanda, and for that I was grateful.

I called Amanda each night, more shocked each time that she was somehow worse than the last time we had spoken. Time went on, and our calls got shorter and shorter. Sometimes I'm quite sure she fell asleep while we talked. Other times, she couldn't even hold the phone. But every day, through the haze of drugs and pain, Amanda asked her parents: "Did Molly carry the torch yet?"

December 27, 2001

Molly,

Just a note to let you know how much you mean to our family. By you carrying the Olympic Torch we feel you are carrying Amanda's spirit with you. Amanda said that you are an inspiration for her, and I know that you have helped Amanda make it this far. She needed someone to share her concerns with and you have filled that role for her at a crucial time in her illness. Our family will forever remember your love and kindness for Amanda.

Our hearts ache because we can't watch you carry the torch in person, but please know we are with you in thought and prayer. You will always have a place in our home and you and your family will be welcome to visit. Please stay in touch with us, and we will contact you if there is any change in Amanda's condition.

Helen Keller once said, "The best and most beautiful things in the world cannot be seen or even touched. They must be felt with the heart." I think Helen Keller would be proud of you.

Our prayers are with you.

Love,
Bernie, Martha, Amanda, Nicholas,
Caroline and William Sherwood.

On December 30, 2001, the Olympic flame arrived in Saratoga Springs, New York, 20 miles south of Glens Falls. I woke up at six a.m., dressed in my Official Torchbearers white warm-up suit and walked downtown in the early morning darkness to meet others who had been chosen to carry the Torch on its journey to Salt Lake City. We boarded a small, private bus and were driven to the outskirts of town, where we sat, waiting for the flame to arrive. When the bus stopped, a man up front broke the silence.

"Congratulations on being selected to carry the Olympic Flame!"

"Thank you," we said in unison.

"You are all here today because someone thought you were inspirational. I'd like everyone to please stand up, say your name and tell us who nominated you and why."

One by one, the people told their stories, and one by one, the stories became more and more emotional.

"My name is Ken Grey, and this is my son's best friend, Devin Wilmot. Devin nominated my son, Billy, to carry the torch while he was being treated for a brain tumor," he said. "Billy was chosen," Ken's voice began to crack, "but he lost his battle just a few months ago at age 12." He put his hand on Devin's shoulder and continued. "Devin and I have been asked to run in Billy's honor."

Could I really be on the same bus with these people? The stories were sad, wonderful and inspirational. I hadn't thought of myself in that way. I was just going through life, playing the hand that I'd been dealt. Is that what they were all doing too?

Next, the woman in the seat across from me stood up.

"My name is Laura Snider. I was a world-class marathon runner but became a victim of domestic violence."

I listened as Laura told her story of abuse. One night, when she and her boyfriend were driving, he told her he wanted to take both of their lives. Then he crashed their car into a tree. Laura suffered multiple broken bones and was told she would never walk again. Now she was about to run with the Olympic Torch and was training to run the Chicago Marathon.

Then it was my turn.

"My name is Molly McMaster and I'm a colon cancer survivor." Hundreds of pictures flashed before my eyes. There was so much to tell. "I was diagnosed on my 23rd birthday in 1999 and wanted to do crazy things to raise awareness of the disease. In the summer of 2000, I in-line skated from Glens Falls to Colorado. Then in November of the same year, I ran the New York City Marathon." I looked at Laura. "And I think you're crazy," I said with a smile. "The marathon was one of the hardest things I've ever chosen to do!" We both laughed.

"I was nominated to carry the Torch by another young colon cancer survivor named Amanda Sherwood Roberts, in Little Rock, Arkansas. Amanda was supposed to be here today, but her cancer has spread. She's not expected to live much longer. I'm running for her this morning."

When I finished, the Olympic tradition began. Each time the bus stopped, one of the runners would disembark and carry the Olympic Flame along the route. We watched through the back window as each torchbearer jogged their distance, passed the glorious flame to the next runner and had their own torch extinguished.

The excitement was unbelievable, but carrying the torch was also bittersweet. I had dreamed of representing the United States on the Women's Olympic Ice Hockey Team. Cancer changed my life. Carrying the Olympic Flame would likely be the closest I would ever get. As I thought about Amanda and how we should have been together for this moment, two young women fighting stupid cancer, I began to let go of my old dream. Amanda and Katie Couric had both planted their seeds, and a new dream was taking root inside of me.

When it was my turn to exit the bus, there was a big surprise and I was overwhelmed with emotion. A sign that said "Good Golly Miss Molly" hung from the side of an RV, and many friends and family members had come out to support me.

I saw many of my friends and hockey teammates, Sergei and some of his teammates, Mom and Dad (wearing his embarrassingly large and fuzzy Russian hat) and Rocky, who had come all the way from Boston with his girlfriend.

I watched the runner coming toward me, wishing Amanda were by my side. He stopped a few feet away from me. I tilted my torch toward his, and as my torch burst into a beautiful flame, I promised myself that I would never stop spreading the message about colon cancer.

Suddenly, I was running. As I turned and waved to the crowd, I was surprised to see a giant picture of Amanda bobbing up and down and moving along with me. Hannah and Angela, Amanda's best friend, were behind the poster, holding her picture high into the air.

That afternoon, Benita Zahn, the WNYT reporter who had interviewed me at the airport before my first visit to Amanda, sent a video clip to NBC in Little Rock so that Amanda could watch me carry the Olympic Flame.

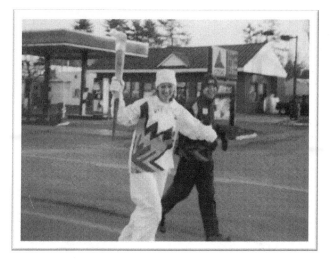

Carrying the Olympic Torch

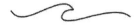

Two days later, on January 1, 2002, Bernie called.

"Hey, Bernie! How are you?" I asked.

"I'm OK," he said softly, but I could hear in his voice that he was not.

"Amanda died today, Molly."

I caught my breath and choked back tears. I knew her death was inevitable, but when I heard Bernie's voice, a tiny part of me still hoped that he was calling to tell me there had been a miracle.

"She waited for you to carry the Torch," he said, "and then she was ready to let go."

"Bernie, I'm so sorry," I said, swallowing my tears. "I love you all."

"We love you too, Sweetie," he said, and hung up the phone.

I put the phone back into its cradle and let my tears fall. It was the first time I had cried for Amanda. I cried for the girl who had lost her battle with colon cancer and for the two children who would grow up without their mother. I cried for Bernie and Martha, who had lost their only daughter; for Nicholas, who had lost his only sister. And I cried for myself, for the friend I had lost, the only friend who knew what I had gone through.

I took a deep breath and wiped the tears from my face, remembering what I had told myself as I had run with the torch. Amanda had been there with me that day and she would never leave. I would carry a part of her with me for the rest of my life.

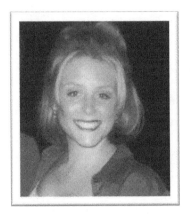

Amanda Sherwood Roberts
Nov. 23, 1974 – Jan. 1, 2002

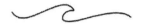

January 11, 2002

Dear Molly:

I was saddened to learn about the recent death of Amanda Sherwood Roberts. I know this is a difficult time for Amanda's family and her many friends.

Your work to raise awareness in regard to colon cancer is a wonderful tribute to Amanda and to your own courage. Your ability to turn your personal battle against the horrible disease into a campaign to help spread awareness and save lives is remarkable. I know that you have done extraordinary things to call attention to this very important issue, including recently carrying the Olympic Torch.

Thank you so much for the vital service you are providing for our nation. Please stay in touch with my office and let me know if there is anything I can do to help you in this important mission.

Sincerely yours,
Hillary Rodham Clinton

20

A COLOSSAL PROJECT

As January of 2002 got under way, Sergei and I were beginning our third year together and putting the finishing touches on our new apartment. I was settling into my new position as Morning Show co-host at the local radio station after moving from the afternoon slot. When *Parade* magazine ran a photo and article about Amanda and me the day after her funeral, my desire to educate the world about colon cancer roared back with a vengeance. There was no reason *anyone* should die of colon cancer. I could not forget my promise to Amanda, or Katie Couric's challenge. My wheels began to turn.

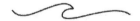

Hello again, Molly!

An aunt and uncle of mine visited today and brought a copy of Parade magazine. They were curious to know if the Molly in the article was <u>MY</u> Molly. Sure enough! There you were with Amanda! You've become quite the celebrity!

Fondly,
Nancy

Each day, I woke up and asked myself a simple question: "What can I do next?" I wanted people to talk about their colons in the same way they talked about having their teeth cleaned. But how could I make that happen? Whatever it was, it had to be big, it had to make people look twice, and it had to educate both young and old.

One morning, it hit me. While hurrying through my morning shower, a picture flashed through my mind. It was one of those giant Slinky toys I used to crawl through as a kid in gym class.

"That's it!" I said aloud. "I'm going to build a giant colon!"

That morning, after my shift at the radio station, I called my brother's girlfriend.

"Aimee, could you possibly meet me and Mom for lunch? I need your medical expertise."

"Are you OK?" she asked.

"Yeah. I'm fine," I said. I just want to bounce my latest crazy idea off of you."

As we sat around a table eating sandwiches, I revealed my newest scheme.

"You know how I've been trying to come up with something ever since Katie Couric's comment when I was on *Today* with Amanda?"

"She told you that if you thought of anything crazy for Colorectal Cancer Awareness Month, she'd have you back on the show." Mom said.

"Right," I said, "and I think I've come up with something crazy that I don't think she'll be able to refuse. It's big and it's out there and I think it will be great!"

Mom and Aimee looked like they were ready to jump out of their skin.

"Will you tell us already?" Mom said.

"I want to build a giant colon!" I said.

"What?" Mom said.

"I want to build a giant colon," I repeated.

"What for?" Aimee asked.

"People could crawl through it and learn about colon cancer. Then hopefully they will start talking about it."

"And learn how easy it is to *not get*," Mom said, already helping to sell my new project. We sat for a few moments in silence, pondering the idea of the great colon beast. What was going through Aimee's mind? As a Nurse Practitioner, she was the first medical professional to hear this plan. Her response was important. Finally, Aimee laughed.

"That's a great idea. What will it be like?" she asked.

"I'm not exactly sure yet," I said. "I'm picturing one of those giant, accordion, Slinky-things we used to crawl through in gym class, but we could show what the inside of the human colon actually looks like. Maybe even show what a tumor looks like."

"You should have a few polyps in there to show how you can remove them before the cancer starts," Mom suggested.

"That's a great idea," I said, jotting notes on my napkin.

"Not to cause trouble, Molly, but there are other diseases of the colon too," Aimee said. "Maybe you should consider putting some of those in as well, so that people understand that if they're having symptoms, it may not necessarily be colon cancer that's causing them."

"Yup, great," I said, still scribbling. "Dad had diverticulitis a long time ago. We could put that in there."

"Sure," Aimee said, "Crohn's disease, diverticulitis, ulcerative colitis. There are quite a few different colon diseases. You should try to get as many in there as you can."

"When Molly first went into the hospital, didn't they ask about Crohn's?" Mom asked.

"I think so," Aimee said. "As for the polyps, you could put both cancerous and non-cancerous in and show that not all polyps necessarily turn into cancer."

"Good stuff," I said, continuing to take notes.

"And it could get worse as you go through," she continued, "starting with normal healthy colon tissue and working its way into non-cancerous polyps, then to cancerous polyps and then worsening tumors."

"Yeah," I said, "And maybe we finish with a bang – stage IV colon cancer at the end, busting out of the colon wall."

"That may be getting a bit graphic," Aimee said.

"What's the entrance going to look like?" Mom interrupted.

"I'd be more worried about the exit," Aimee said through laughter.

"Could you get me some pictures?" I asked Aimee.

"I'll see if the gastro docs will give me some, but I'm sure we can find a few of them online too."

"How big are you planning to make this thing?" Mom asked.

"I want people to crawl through it, so not too tall, but I'd definitely like it to be as long as possible --- not a five-foot long tube where they can see the other end. I want it to be, well, colonesque."

"*Colonesque*?" Mom repeated.

"I really want people to feel like they're inside a colon, like they're making the real journey, you know?"

"Molly," Mom said, laughing again, "You're too much."

"Does that mean you'd have to 'prep' before you crawl through?" Aimee asked with a chuckle.

"Sure," I played along.

"In case the prep hasn't done its job, everyone should wear rubber suits," Mom said, adding to the brainstorm.

"You could be a human colonoscope," Aimee spit out between tears and laughter, "and wear one of those hiking headlamps."

The three of us laughed and joked. People in the restaurant stopped their lunch to listen to us. This was going to be a fun project.

That night, Aimee sent an email with a few colonoscopy pictures and a link to a real colonoscopy video. "I don't mean to be a pain in the ass," Aimee wrote, "but what about hemorrhoids?"

Just a few days later, on January 10, 2002, I went to Adirondack Scenic Inc. (now called Adirondack Studios), a company that builds Broadway musical sets, amusement park pieces and creates all kinds of imaginative objects. Maggie, from Glens Falls Hospital's Cancer Prevention and Early Detection Department joined me, along with Carl, the company's sales manager, and a few of the company's designers and engineers. We sat around a large table and discussed my proposal.

"Alright, Molly," Carl said. "Since no one seems to believe me when I tell them what you're looking for, could you explain again?"

"Sure," I said. "I want to build a giant colon!" Everyone laughed.

"So, Carl, you *were* telling the truth," joked Randy, senior art director at Adirondack Scenic.

"I was diagnosed with colon cancer on my 23rd birthday." Around the table, everyone seemed to get a little bit tense.

"Is everything OK now?" Randy asked.

"Yup," I continued, hoping to take the edge off. "Everything's fine. My doctor is pretty sure they removed everything during surgery, but I went through chemo just in case."

"OK," Randy said, getting back to business. "What do you picture?"

"I want to be able to crawl through it."

"Not walk through?" Carl asked. "I have to tell you that with my knees I probably wouldn't be crawling through it."

"I want everyone to know about colon cancer, but I really want to target kids and younger adults since the older population seems to be pretty well covered when it comes to education." I thought back to a recent conversation I had with a woman from the American Cancer Society. She had explained that because I "didn't fall within their statistics," I would not be allowed to speak for or represent them in any educational projects. I argued with her. I told her Amanda's story and my story. I even pulled up my shirt to show her my scar. I had left the room in tears, and I vowed that I would never exclude anyone, especially younger people, from my projects to raise awareness.

"I want to target the people who don't fall within the normal statistics," I said.

Randy scribbled on a piece of paper. "But you do want adults who are willing to brave the giant colon to be able to crawl through, so we should probably make it tall enough for a six-foot-tall man to sit up inside. But what about those people like Carl who don't want to or can't crawl through it?"

"Honestly," I said, "I haven't gotten that far."

"What about windows or viewing ports in the top? That would take care of the lighting problem too," Carl said.

"That would be good," I agreed.

"How about length? Is 10 feet long enough?" Randy asked.

"I'd like it to be as long as possible, within what we can afford. I'd like it to turn or zigzag, so you can't see out the other end as you're crawling through."

"OK," Randy continued scribbling.

For an hour, we dickered about lengths and widths, materials and logistics while Randy took pages and pages of notes.

"Let's give our designer here some time and get together again in a week," Carl finally said.

When I got home, I called Amanda's cousin, Hannah.

"You want to build a *what?*" she asked.

"A giant colon!"

"OK," she said with a laugh but without argument. "We can do this. Send me all the information you have so far. How much will it cost? Who is your target audience? What is it exactly and how will it be built? List all the basics and we'll turn it into a fundraising proposal." Grateful that we could use Hannah's fundraising expertise to raise more awareness of colon cancer, I immediately started a list.

As Hannah worked on the proposal for what she had cleverly named the Colossal Colon, I could hardly wait for my next meeting at Adirondack Scenic. Again, our crew sat around the table.

"Here's what we've come up with," Randy began. He handed Maggie and me a large drawing showing a winding, u-shaped colon model with a curtain backdrop behind it. On the backdrop, a sign said, "Colossal Colon," and on both sides of the colon there were tables where volunteers would hand out information. It was exactly what I wanted!

"That's the basic design," Randy said. "If there's anything you don't like, just let us know." He handed us each another sheet of paper. "And these are our options on how to build it." There were three different design options with an estimated cost for each.

"The first choice we have is an inflatable colon," Randy explained. "It's somewhat-like the Bouncy Bounce at the county fair --- same material and concept. It's going to be the cheapest to build, easy to store and move, and easy to deal with in general. The drawback is that it won't be very realistic, almost cartoony, and you'll need an electric fan to keep it up, which means that you'll need a power source or generator wherever you are."

Maggie and I both nodded.

"The second choice is a little bit more realistic. We would start with a metal frame and put soft foam and fabric over that. It will be somewhat flexible and more realistic but won't be able to break apart, which is something you had told Carl you wanted to do so you could take individual pieces into schools if you have a speaking engagement, right?"

"Right," I answered.

"It will also be bulky and pretty hard to clean."

We nodded again and Randy continued. "The final colon design that we've come up with is the most realistic of all, but also the most expensive. It will also be pretty bulky but can be taken apart. For that one, we would begin with a wooden frame and then spray a polyurethane foam over it, before we carve it into the shape we want. Then we paint over that and finish with a clear and shiny top coat."

When Randy finished explaining and I had digested the estimated costs, we all shook hands.

"We'll get back to you when we've raised the money."

"You want it by the beginning of March, right?" Carl asked.

"Yes," I said.

"We're probably going to need confirmation by February 1 in order to finish it on time then. Keep me posted. This is a pretty interesting project."

In the parking lot, Maggie and I discussed the proposed designs. We both nixed the first design, the inflatable colon. We liked the second one, but the third was definitely the most realistic option.

"If we can raise the money for the second one they showed us, there's no reason we shouldn't be able to raise a few thousand more and get the best one, right?" I said.

"That's what I was thinking," she said, getting into her car.

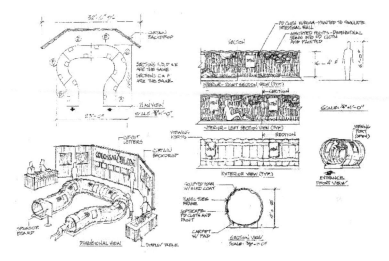

Adirondack Scenic Inc., Colossal Colon Design

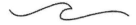

On the ride home, I couldn't stop thinking about the Colossal Colon. How on earth would we make it happen? No one could resist a giant colon, especially Katie Couric, but we had to raise $60,000. It was January 16. Carl said they needed confirmation by February 1 in order to create it by March, which was National Colorectal Cancer Awareness Month. We only had 15 days. It was going to take a miracle.

I called Hannah and told her about the three different colon choices and the three different prices.

"We might as well go ahead and just raise enough money for the best one," I said.

"OK!" she said enthusiastically. "This project is really going to get people talking!"

Two days later, we finished the proposal together, with the title blazing across the top, "Colossal Colon Corporate Proposal." I couldn't help but laugh as I made copies for the pharmacist at my cancer center, who promised to hand them directly to oncology drug reps. I also had a copy for the American Cancer Society representatives with whom I was planning to meet that afternoon.

Rolling to Recovery had raised $60,000, one-third of which I had given to the American Cancer Society. I had asked them not to use it until I had approved an educational project, and now that I had one, my hope was that they would put the money into the Colossal Colon. It would be a great educational tool. If they gave the money, not only could they put their name on it, but they could also use it at any events they chose.

As I prepared for my meeting with the Cancer Society representatives, one sentence kept echoing in my head: "You don't fall within our statistics." The more I replayed it, the angrier I became. I was about to meet with the same people and ask for money that I had raised in the first place. Unfortunately, I knew they might be our only hope.

That afternoon, I pleaded my case.

"Molly, we're going to have to speak with our state office before we can give you an answer," one of the representatives said. "Are you available for a conference call?" I thought they would have been thrilled with such an exciting, new idea, but I might as well have asked if I could have a bake sale. We scheduled a call, and the meeting was over.

Each day, Hannah and I chatted about all the things we could do with the Colossal Colon.

"When we get this thing built, we can send it touring all over the country!" When I said the words, I was completely serious, picturing our giant colon traveling around in a U-Haul.

We sent more fundraising proposals to various charities, and a week after my first meeting, I sat in on a conference call with the New York State office of the American Cancer Society.

"We're going to have to speak with the national level about this," they told me. "Let's set up another conference call."

We seemed to be driving down a dead-end road. They still didn't show much excitement about the Colossal Colon, and I still hadn't convinced them that young people could be the best and most energetic educators. Meanwhile, rejection letters began to arrive in response to our grant proposals. Hope was dwindling.

Then, on January 25, I met a drug rep from Pharmacia Corporation who wanted to take me to lunch and talk about the Colossal Colon.

"What colon cancer drug does Pharmacia make?" I asked over sushi, curious to know why they were interested in giving money.

"We make Camptosar," she said. That was one of the drugs that Marie had been on. "It's used as first-line therapy for treatment of patients with advanced stages of colon or rectal cancer, along with 5-FU and leucovorin."

I told her about my diagnosis and my "crazy things" to raise awareness. I told her about Amanda and my promise, the *Today* show and Katie's challenge.

"Pharmacia is definitely interested in helping out," she said. "I'll have to speak with the higher-ups, of course. But I'll get back to you."

After our lunch, there was a glimmer of hope that the Colossal Colon might happen.

On January 30, when I had given up on hearing from Pharmacia, my cell phone rang.

"My name is Peg. I'm with Roche Pharmaceuticals. I got your proposal for the Colossal Colon the other day and was hoping I could speak with you about it."

"Absolutely. What can I tell you?"

"Well, first, let me tell you that Roche is very interested in getting involved."

"That's great," I said.

"And second," she said, "I thought you'd like to know that the rep who gave your proposal to me said that the pharmacist at your hospital is quite sure that you'll do well. What was it he said? I think it was 'You *want* to get on board for this. This girl *will* get publicity.'" We both laughed.

"This is all over a promise that I made to a friend who died recently of colon cancer at age 27," I said. "My friend and I were on the *Today* show and Katie Couric told me that if I could come up with anything crazy for National Colorectal Cancer Awareness Month, she would have me on the show again."

"So, if the Colossal Colon is built, are you going to take it on the show?" she asked.

"Absolutely! Assuming Katie will still have us."

Peg and I spoke for about 10 minutes. The next morning, she gave me unofficial confirmation that Roche would give us half of the money toward the project. We were halfway there, but time was running out.

Later that morning, Hannah and I had another conference call with the American Cancer Society, but this time it was with the national office and there were six people representing ACS.

"Molly, can you explain your idea to us again?"

"Sure," I began with a sigh, growing tired of explaining to the same people over and over again why the Colossal Colon was such an awesome idea. The fact was, it could educate thousands of people. Wasn't that what mattered?

By the end of the call, I was near tears. They needed to discuss it further and asked to set up yet another conference call.

Hannah and I reluctantly agreed, telling them that we absolutely needed an answer by Monday, just a few days away.

When we hung up, Hannah and I discussed our options.

"You know, we can always wait until next year," Hannah said. She was much more patient than I. "Or, we could build it during another month. It doesn't have to be March, you know. That's not the only month that people get colon cancer."

That night, I couldn't sleep. We had a commitment from Roche for half the money, and private donations amounted to another $5,000 or so. We were so close, but with ACS dragging their heels, our time might run out.

When I did open my eyes the next day, I felt like a bomb had gone off inside my head. I called in sick and fell back into a deep sleep. I finally peeled the covers back around 10 a.m., and clutching a box of tissues, stumbled into our home office to check my email.

It was February 1, the day Carl needed to know if we had raised the money. Failure rested heavily on my mind, adding to the head cold I had picked up overnight. It had been a great idea --- an *amazing* idea. Why couldn't ACS see that?

The phone rang.

"Hi, Molly. My name is Janine."

"And I'm Sherry," a second woman said. "We're from the Cancer Research Foundation of America. We're calling because we heard about the Colossal Colon and we think it's a fabulous idea! We were hoping you might let us borrow it sometime, if that's possible."

"Oh, wow. Um, I'd love to." I cleared my throat. "But at this point it doesn't look like it's going to happen. We're having trouble getting the money together. Roche has offered half, but we have a ways to go. You'd be surprised how much a 40-foot colon costs," I joked.

"Oh. That's too bad. It's a really great idea. Please let us know if we can do anything."

"Thanks."

I hung up the phone and stared at the computer screen. My stomach churned, I was sniffling and I felt lightheaded. How many people would we reach with the Colossal Colon? Hundreds? Thousands? Maybe even millions.

Twenty minutes later, the phone rang again.

"It's Janine and Sherry again, from the Cancer Research Foundation of America."

"Couldn't get enough of me the first time, huh?" They laughed.

"We would like to match Roche's financial contribution if you'll give us the opportunity to take the Colossal Colon on a national tour next year."

"You're kidding!" I stood up from the chair and jumped up and down. This was our miracle, and just in the nick of time.

That evening, Sergei and I celebrated the Colossal Colon with a bottle of wine.

"Congratulations, Baby!" he said. "Cheers!" He clinked his glass with mine.

"Thanks! I still can't believe it's going to happen." I looked at the clock.

"Eleven, Eleven," I said. "Make a wish."

"What *are* you going to wish for?" Sergei asked.

"You know I can't tell you that."

21

KEEPING MY PROMISE

On February 6, the March issue of *Self* magazine hit the stands, and I was inside the front cover in the editor's column, running with the Olympic Torch. It was surreal. Someone out there would get a colonoscopy because I talked about the embarrassing stuff no one else wanted to talk about. It almost made me think that I was supposed to get this disease.

Meanwhile, Maggie and I were working with Adirondack Scenic. She was in charge of the diseases on the interior of the colon model. The only interior of a colon I'd seen was my own, on a video screen during my last colonoscopy.

Maggie met with gastroenterologists at Glens Falls Hospital. She got real colonoscopy footage and photos and brought them to Adirondack Scenic. We visited a couple times a week and watched the Colossal Colon transform from what looked like a wooden skeleton of a dinosaur, to a giant worm and then a true piece of art. The engineers and artists at Adirondack Scenic worked overtime to get the job done on time.

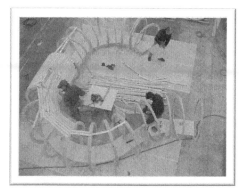

Colossal Colon Frame - Adirondack Scenic Inc.

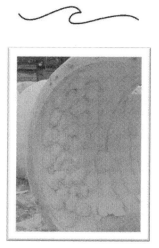

Carving Polyposis - Adirondack Scenic Inc.

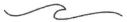

I celebrated my 26th birthday with a family dinner and a few days later I had my three-year checkup, a CT scan and chest X-ray, which were all good. Then, in late February, I received confirmation that the Aviation Mall in nearby Queensbury would have a vacant store available to display the Colossal Colon for the month of March. Local newspapers and news stations reported that "McMaster was planning something BIG for Colorectal Cancer Awareness Month." They took pictures and filmed the building process.

On March 1, we launched the Cool Rock Colossal Colon Contest on our morning radio show. Each day I repeated a new colon cancer "factoid" during the show. For example: "Colon cancer is one of the only forms of cancer you can get rid of before it even starts, just by removing the polyp." To enter the contest, listeners were asked to call in and repeat the "factoid." At the end of the month, our contestants would meet us at the mall for a live radio broadcast. They would crawl through the Colossal Colon, pick a "polyp," which was actually a red balloon, and win a prize.

People were learning about their colons, tests for colon cancer and the screening colonoscopy. More importantly, people were talking about their colons, which was the first step in getting them to talk to their doctors and get screened.

On March 6, 2002, Adirondack Scenic delivered the Colossal Colon to the Aviation Mall, its home for National Colorectal Cancer Awareness Month. It took just over a month to build it, but everyone involved knew that every second was worth it.

The Colossal Colon proudly stood 40-feet long and four-feet tall and displayed everything from healthy colon tissue to colon polyps and various stages of cancer, as well as diverticulosis, Crohn's Disease, ulcerative colitis and even hemorrhoids, as Aimee had suggested. The navy blue, glitter-star backdrop offered a hint of glitzy Hollywood, and "For Amanda" was written inconspicuously on the side of the colon. I knew she would have been proud.

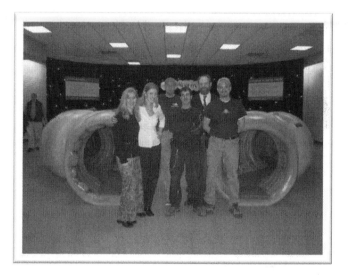

Opening Day at Aviation Mall

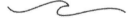

The first day the Colossal Colon was open to visitors, newspaper photographers and reporters were there for most of the day. I did a live interview with Benita Zahn from WNYT, and the crowd began to pour in.

The second day, *The Post-Star,* the newspaper that ran my Rolling to Recovery journal as a column, ran a half-page color photo that showed me crawling through the colon.

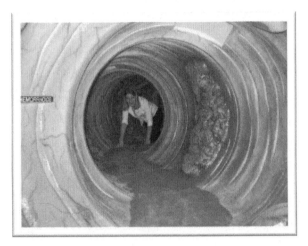

Crawling Through the Colossal Colon

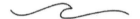

Throughout the month of March, hundreds of people came to see the Colossal Colon. Mom, Maggie and I, and our many volunteers, took turns colon-sitting.

Some people walked by the retail space pretending nothing was there. Others rushed in saying "Oh! I saw this in the paper!" or "I watched this on TV!" Some people made rude jokes. There were visitors who said it was disgusting and others who thought the colon was turning a serious disease into a joke. Others stopped and stared but wouldn't enter the store, perhaps afraid they might get sucked into the giant colon. But the joke was on them because I knew that every single person would go home that night, sit at the dinner table and talk about what they saw at the mall. They would start a conversation about colon cancer and that was the first step to getting screened.

My favorite reaction came from a boy who was about seven years old. He stopped, looked wide-eyed at the colon, then crossed his arms and said boldly, "I'm *not* going in there!"

When his parents entered the store, he followed slowly and far behind them. Mom and Dad circled the outside of the colon and looked in the windows.

"You sure you don't want to go in?" his father asked.

"*No way*," the boy said, retreating to safety outside the entrance. Then they all left.

But 30 minutes later they were back, leading the boy by the hand. "We'll buy you some candy if you just crawl through once," the mother bribed.

The boy pursed his lips tightly and shook his head.

"OK," she said, removing her shoes. "I'm going through."

"*No!*" he yelled and grabbed her hand, fearing she would be swallowed up by the huge colon beast.

"You can come too," she said.

"*No!*"

Again, he tried to pull her back, to save her from being eaten alive, but it was too late. She was on her knees and crawling through.

The boy ran to the exit, watching intently for his mother to appear. When she emerged, he grabbed her hand and pulled her out of the store.

They passed by a few more times that afternoon, and each time I heard Mom or Dad offer him a new bribe.

The next afternoon, they appeared again, but this time the youngster slowly walked up to the colon with his mother and took off his shoes. Together they knelt and entered the Colossal Colon without a word.

When they came out the other end, the boy asked shyly, "Can I go through again?"

"Of course," his mother said, winking at Mom and me. As he entered the colon over and over again, his mother turned to my Mom. "I don't know what happened," she said. "Yesterday, he wouldn't go through it to save his own life, but today when he got home from school he asked if we could go to the mall. He said he wanted to crawl through the Colossal Colon."

"Maybe he wants to be a gastroenterologist," I joked.

In mid-March, we got the news we'd all been waiting for. The *Today* show wanted the Colossal Colon.

I emailed Nancy to let her know that I was taking my big colon to the city. I was hoping we could finally meet each other. But her reply was not what I expected.

Molly, I'm so proud of you, and I know Amanda is too! It's about time Katie took notice again! You will be wonderful on the Today show, and I will be watching, but won't be able to make it into the city this time. My illness is taking over, and I have accepted my fate. I'm in stage IV now, and I know that my time will be soon. Please don't feel sorry for me, as this was God's intention for me.

I so wanted to meet you and take you to lunch at Tavern on the Green — after all, it's practically a crime that you've never been there — but I won't be able to. I'm sending you a check, and I want you to promise me that you and Sergei will have a big lunch. Don't say no, because I'm mailing it anyway. I really wanted to be able to take you myself, but this will have to do.

Good luck on the show. I know that you will be fabulous!

Love,
Nancy

On March 20, 2002, Katie Couric made good on her promise and stood in the rain under a white tent in Rockefeller Plaza with me, the Colossal Colon and Hannah, who was representing her cousin Amanda.

"March is National Colorectal Cancer Awareness Month," Katie began. "We want to focus on the second leading cancer killer in this country, colorectal cancer. We first met Molly McMaster in November of last year."

Katie then told the story of Amanda's illness and the Olympic Torch.

"Now, in honor of Amanda Sherwood Roberts and National Colorectal Cancer Awareness Month, Molly McMaster is here with Amanda's cousin, Hannah, and a 40-foot long Colossal Colon, which Molly conceived as a way to raise awareness about colon cancer screening and prevention."

Hannah and I talked about the miracle of raising money to build the colon and how it was dedicated to the memory of Amanda. Then, with the cameras rolling and people watching on their televisions across the country, Hannah took them on a tour through the Colossal Colon.

That afternoon, Sergei and I took a cab in the rain to Tavern on the Green. Crystal chandeliers lit the Terrace Room where we were seated, and windows all around allowed us to watch the raindrops spatter the glass and sparkle like a million stars. Nancy should have been there.

After lunch, as we stood in the lobby waiting for the drizzle to subside. A man approached me.

"Hey, weren't you on TV this morning? With Katie Couric and a giant colon?"

"Yeah," I smiled.

"I recognized your shirt," he said, looking at the words "I crawled through the Colossal Colon" on the back of my outfit.

"Clever. Great job! Was that thing your idea?"

"Yeah," I said again, blushing.

"My mother died of colon cancer," he said. "I'm going in for my colonoscopy soon. Thank you for what you're doing."

"Thank you for getting screened," I said.

When I arrived home from New York City and the *Today* show interview, Don Coyote, a cartoon commentator in *The Post-Star* newspaper, made his opinion about the Colossal Colon known too.

"I hurt my back shoveling this stupid snow. My car died. I lost my retirement money in the Enron Scandal. And I'm in last place in the NCAA office pool. This is turning out to be one Colossal Colon of a day."

With the now nationally known Colossal Colon back at the Aviation Mall, more people were visiting than ever. I told my story to school groups, asking them to talk to their parents about symptoms and family history. I talked strangers into getting their first colonoscopies.

Along with many volunteers, I spent the entire month talking about colorectal cancer. I was feeling a passion that until that point, I had only felt when I was on the ice.

A few months after the Colossal Colon had left the mall and was safely in storage, awaiting our national tour in 2003, I got a call from Cathy, a nurse from the GI Center at Glens Falls Hospital. She had been a volunteer at the mall.

"I have a story that I wanted you to hear," she said. "An older gentleman recently came in for his colonoscopy and told us that you talked him into having it while the Colossal Colon was at the mall."

"Really? Who was he?" I had talked with so many people. I couldn't possibly pinpoint one particular person.

"He said you had mentioned a friend of yours in New Jersey who never got her colonoscopy, and now she is losing her fight."

I immediately remembered the man. After the Colossal Colon made her debut on national television and was back at the mall, I saw an older man standing at the edge of the store, hesitating to come in.

"We only bite on Tuesdays," I told him, and he laughed. "Would you like to crawl through our colon?"

"No. No. That's OK. I'm too old to be crawling through."

"There are windows in the top," I said. "You're more than welcome to have a look around.

At that, he took a few steps into the store. "Have you gotten your colonoscopy yet?" I asked. He was startled by my bluntness, but he was definitely over age 50, and for me, this had become a perfectly normal conversation.

"I'm not getting that thing," he said, looking disgusted.

"Oh, come on," I said. "It's not that bad. I've had two of them. The worst part is the prep you have to drink the night before. Ask anyone."

He didn't seem amused but walked around the outside of the colon and peeked inside through the windows.

"You're that girl who skated across the country, aren't you?" It was a question I had heard often in the past few years.

"Yup. That's me," I said. "I'm a colon cancer survivor, and I'm raising awareness so that other people don't have to go through what I did."

"I think you're really great," he said.

"Thanks," I said. "But why haven't you had your colonoscopy? That's why I do these things, you know, to teach people about the symptoms and get them screened."

"I'm sure I'm fine," he said. "I don't have any of those symptoms."

"Did you know that the most common symptom of colon cancer is no symptom at all?" I said, not missing a beat. "That's why people with average risk factors have to get their colonoscopies when they turn 50."

"I've been healthy all my life," he said. "Ain't nothing wrong with me now."

"You're probably right, but I have a friend who would tell you differently."

"Who's that?" he asked.

"My friend Nancy lives in New Jersey," I said. "She told me that her husband has been getting colonoscopies every five years since he was 40."

"So?"

"So, she never got one."

"What happened to her?" he asked. I knew I had to be blunt.

"She has stage IV colon cancer now. Her doctor doesn't expect her to live much longer," I said. "I can't tell you how many times she's told me that she wished she'd gotten a colonoscopy sooner."

"How old is she?" he asked.

"She's in her early sixties." The man looked at me wide-eyed.

"Best of luck to you," he said, and he left the store.

Cathy's voice brought me back to our phone conversation.

"I just had to tell you this story. When he came in to get screened, he was diagnosed with very early stage colon cancer."

I was stunned. "Molly," she said, "you saved that man's life. He had it removed and won't even need chemo. He's going to be fine."

Tears rolled down my cheeks. I had found what I had been chosen to do and I was keeping my promise to Amanda.

22

COCO HITS THE ROAD

I loved my job in radio, but I had an obligation to fulfill, so I left the station to prepare for the Colossal Colon's 20-city national tour, presented by the Cancer Research & Prevention Foundation (formerly the Cancer Prevention Foundation of America) and sponsored by Roche.

Leading up to the tour, Hannah and I were invited to attend the annual planning meeting for National Colorectal Cancer Awareness Month in Alexandria, Virginia. We were beyond excited to join the other 50 partnering organizations and couldn't wait to share a few ideas, but after a morning of meetings and brainstorming sessions, we were surprised and happy to find that they were already embracing the idea of educating younger people. We didn't have to convince anyone. The organizations had collectively talked about getting into schools to educate kids about symptoms, risk factors and family history of colorectal cancer. The thought was that those kids would then speak with their parents and educate them as well.

Hannah and I didn't want to compete with other organizations. We needed to fill a void. Over lunch, we discussed our soon-to-be-formed nonprofit, and by the time our meal was over, our vision was clearer than it had ever been. We needed to stick with what we knew, what no one else was doing, and quite frankly, what we were good at. Our nonprofit would be formed to do "crazy things" to raise awareness of colorectal cancer, especially in younger people.

On my last day at the radio station before leaving for the tour, I got a call from a reporter at *The Post-Star*.

"I have some good news for you," she said. "Glens Falls Hospital has reported that the number of colonoscopies has gone up locally by 30 percent. I spoke with a few of the nurses and doctors in the GI Center. They're giving you some of the credit."

"Seriously?"

"Yes. I was hoping I could get a comment from you."

Thirty percent? I was stunned.

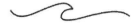

The Colossal Colon, or CoCo, as we had affectionately started calling her, was a huge success in my hometown, but it was time to find out how the rest of the country would receive her. On February 19, 2003, exactly four years from the day I was told that I had colon cancer, CoCo opened her 20-city national tour in Chapel Hill, North Carolina in the middle of an unexpected snowstorm.

2003 Colossal Colon Tour Schedule

Chapel Hill: Feb 19-22	**San Francisco:** Jun 25-28
Washington, D.C.: Mar 5-8	**Seattle:** Jul 9-12
Atlanta: Mar 19-22	**Denver:** Jul 23-26
Miami: Apr 2-5	**Minneapolis:** Aug 6-9
Little Rock: Apr 16-19	**St Louis:** Aug 20-23
Dallas: Apr 23-26	**Detroit:** Sep 3-6
Houston: May 7-10	**Cleveland:** Sep 17-20
Chicago: May 21-24	**Philadelphia:** Oct 1-4
Phoenix: Jun 11-14	**Boston:** Oct 15-18
Los Angeles: Jun 18-21	**New York:** Oct 29- Nov. 1

I left my hotel room early that morning and walked across the UNC-Chapel Hill campus on the icy brick walkway. I had a napkin in my hand, with black scribbling on it that resembled a map. After a few turns, I saw a glistening white tent in the distance. My stomach fluttered. This was it. This was what the past year was all about. The Cancer Research and Prevention Foundation had designed a 10-station exhibit around the Colossal Colon, and I was about to see it for the first time. I veered off the brick walkway, too excited to follow the winding path, and the icy cold seeped through my shoes.

As I hurried to the tent, bright purple signs came into focus. "Check Your Insides Out," a sign said in purple curly font above the doorway. I stepped inside. My mouth fell open. On my right was a fluorescent green welcome station where two women stood in windows that looked like ticket booths for a carnival ride. They were handing out "passports" for the Colossal Colon's national tour.

Ahead, there was an enormous flat screen monitor and an electric green game show set. Flashing lights beckoned contestants to test their colon knowledge by buzzing in and answering into the microphone.

A few steps away, I saw a large purple wall with an outline of a human body from the head to the knees. Inside the outline was a colorful map of the digestive tract, with buttons spaced neatly throughout. I pressed the first button in the mouth of the body, and twinkling yellow lights flashed on a path from the mouth and down the throat. Another yellow light glowed next to the word "Mouth," and the text told what happens when we chew our food. I pushed the next button and the esophagus and the light next to its information flashed green. I pushed each button until everything was flashing a different color, right down to the aqua-colored, flashing anus. I laughed.

A few more steps ahead, there were close-up pictures of CoCo and three videos. The first showed an interview I had done on my couch a few months prior, the second video was about the Colossal Colon's construction, and the third showed the finished CoCo and what it was like to be inside.

As I made my way to the back of the tent, I was taken aback by a large photo of Amanda smiling down at me. It was the same photo she had chosen for her own obituary, but it was ten feet tall. Under her picture was a letter to Colossal Colon visitors from her friends and family, asking them to learn the symptoms of colorectal cancer and to be persistent with their doctors if they have unexplained symptoms. I stopped reading when I realized that chairs and a podium were being set up around me. Preparations for our first press conference were underway. I continued my tour.

CoCo, the star of the show, was in the back of the tent, behind Amanda, but I kept walking to station number six, where there was a bright orange wall with text about colorectal cancer screening. There, behind a dark curtain, in a private viewing area, visitors could watch a video of a man having an actual colonoscopy. They could also see a real colonoscope, the tool a gastroenterologist uses to perform a colonoscopy. On another wall, nine monitors played videos of cancer survivors telling their stories.

Then I turned and discovered a giant roll of paper hanging from a spool. "Messages of Hope," it said above the spool. People had already written notes. Right in the middle, there was a note to me:

Molly, what an outrageous idea that gets everyone's attention! Godspeed with the spread of knowledge!

To the left of the spool was a yellow wall with a picture of broccoli and the words "good health." Diet and exercise were the lessons at station nine.

At station 10, near the exit, a volunteer waited for visitors to check out and sign the pledge on their passport, promising to get screened.

As I stepped back outside, I had butterflies in my stomach and tears in my eyes. It was hard to digest the fact that this had all come from a crazy idea I'd had one morning while in the shower.

When it was time for the press conference to launch CoCo's national tour, cameras rolled in and reporters and guests took their seats.

Carolyn "Bo" Aldege, president and founder of the Cancer Research and Prevention Foundation, kicked it off. A doctor went up to the podium, a survivor was introduced and then it was my turn at the microphone and my palms were sweaty with nervousness.

My talk began with my symptoms in Colorado and being misdiagnosed. I told them about the emergency room, the surgery and my 23rd birthday, the day I found out that I had colon cancer. The more I talked, the easier the words came. I pushed on, telling the audience and reporters about Rolling to Recovery, meeting Amanda, and my promise to her to continue raising awareness. That's when it began to get hard. I tried to hold back tears, but as I talked about losing my friend to colon cancer, with cameras rolling, I broke down and cried.

When I stepped away from the microphone, still wiping tears, I was presented with a birthday cake to celebrate 27 years of life and four years cancer-free.

After a few hours passed and many visitors had come through, I made another lap around the tent, still pinching myself. Then I received the best gift ever.

"Surprise!" Mom, Dad and Sergei said in unison.

"Happy Birthday!" Sergei said, giving me a kiss.

After four days of colon awareness in Chapel Hill, we closed our "test site" on such a high, I almost believed that we really were saving the world. I couldn't begin to imagine the ups and downs that I would encounter over the next nine months.

Two weeks later, we opened in Freedom Plaza in Washington, D.C. The first night, when I turned on CNN in my hotel room, I was ecstatic to find a blurb about the Colossal Colon tour running on the ticker at the bottom of the screen. CoCo made Yahoo's top 10 page that day too. Our project was working. The Colossal Colon was all over the news.

But by the time we reached Robert W. Woodruff Park in Atlanta, George W. Bush had ordered an invasion of Iraq and we were in a virtual media blackout. It was a scary time in the world, but like the light bulb moment I had after 9/11, I knew that people would still die of colorectal cancer. Life would go on. While the media was a huge vehicle for us to get our message out to millions of people, this made our one-on-one interaction much more important. Nothing compared to talking with someone who just happened to be walking by and was brave enough to come inside. Nothing compared to seeing kids crawl through the Colossal Colon and ask questions. Nothing compared to speaking with homeless veterans who didn't know that they could seek treatment from the Veterans Administration. And, of course, nothing compared to the looks on people's faces when I told them that I was a survivor of colon cancer, diagnosed on my 23rd birthday. Jaws dropped. Tears spilled. There were hugs. It was an absolutely incredible phenomenon.

When CoCo reached Miami, her fourth stop, the tent was situated on South Beach.

"My colon is at the beach!" I excitedly told anyone who would listen. But it was obvious from the blank stares of the bikini-clad beach-goers that CoCo was going to be a tough sell.

We went through our press conference again. After my talk, the media interviewed a few of us, and as I answered my last question, I did a double take as I saw a man emerging from the Colossal Colon, at the exit with the giant hemorrhoids. It was Dave Barry, the syndicated humor columnist from the Miami Herald. I wanted to run over and tell him that I had just finished one of his books, that I loved his column and thought he was fabulous. I wanted to hear him tell jokes about CoCo, But I was star-struck and couldn't bring myself to walk over. Then, just as I was about to walk the other way, Bo said "Molly, come over and meet Dave Barry."

My face went red and I could barely speak.

"Hi," he said. "Was this thing your idea?"

"Yes," I said, and let out a nervous laugh.

"Molly, let's get your picture with Dave. Is that OK, Dave?" Bo said.

"Right here in the hemorrhoids," I laughed again.

"Perfect," he said, and we knelt together for a photo.

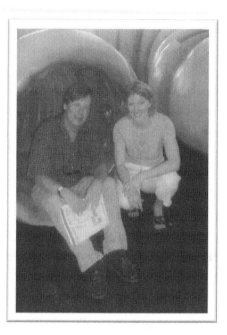

Dave Barry and Me

Miami was a tough sell indeed, but when we opened two weeks later in Amanda's hometown, at the Little Rock River Market Pavilion, there was no shortage of colon lovers. During the press conference, the Arkansas

Secretary of State spoke and made a proclamation, and then Amanda's father, Bernie, made his way to the podium, walking past Amanda's mother and Amanda's two young children. He passed Amanda's aunts, uncles and cousins, and many of her friends, before reaching the microphone to tell her story. Bernie told how Amanda had been pregnant when her symptoms began, and how her doctor had, at first, blamed the symptoms on her pregnancy. He told the crowd about the nurse who informed her of her negative test results, and how she didn't mention that if the test was negative, the doctor wanted Amanda to have a colonoscopy.

"I think my doctor said I'm supposed to get some sort of colonoscope or something like that if it was negative," Amanda had said to her nurse.

"Don't worry, Honey," the nurse had replied. "Surely it will go away."

As I heard the story again, I recalled my own visits with my doctor. She had also been calm and reassuring. Because she was so certain that there was nothing wrong, I thought I was crazy. I was angry all over again.

Bernie continued the story. He told about Amanda's doctor catching the mistake, ordering a colonoscopy and eventually diagnosing her with stage III colon cancer.

I felt angry tears pooling in my eyes and looked away from Amanda's father as he stood in front of the crowd and told them how he lost his only daughter to a monster called colon cancer. I glanced over the standing-room-only crowd and felt comforted. We were all crying together.

It was an exhausting week in Little Rock, physically and emotionally. I felt close to Amanda when I shared

CoCo with the family members and friends who came in droves to volunteer and share her story. Closing our doors was bittersweet, and as I sat in the airport and reflected on the week, I silently questioned myself again. Were we really making a difference? Was CoCo educating people? Was I really keeping my promise to Amanda?

While at the airport gate waiting for my flight, a man dropped a newspaper down on the seat next to me and walked away. I picked it up and scanned the headlines before turning the page to see Dave Barry's smiling face next to a title that made me nearly spit out my coffee.

"GI Journey:
Touring a giant colon and living to tell about it."

BY DAVE BARRY

So there I was, on hands and knees, crawling through a 40-foot long, four-foot-high, human colon.

It wasn't a real colon, of course. No human has a colon that size, except maybe Marlon Brando, and I'm sure he has security people to prevent media access.

No, this was a replica. It's called the Colossal Colon, and I'm not making it up. It was conceived of by a 26-year-old cancer survivor named Molly McMaster as a way to get people to talk about their colons. This is a topic that most people don't even like to THINK about. I sure don't, and I bet you don't. But if you never talk to your doctor about your colon, you might never get screened for colon cancer - the second leading cause of cancer

*death, though it's preventable - and you could die,
and* THEN *think how you'd feel.*

*That's the idea behind the Colossal
Colon, which is currently traveling around the
nation on a 20-city tour (to see if it's coming to your
area, check ColossalColon.com). I caught up with
the colon in South Beach, a part of Miami Beach
known for sophistication and glamour. You can
barely swing your arms there without striking an
international supermodel, or a Rolling Stone, or, at
the bare minimum, a Baldwin brother. I felt that
the Colossal Colon fit right in.*

*The colon was set up inside an air-
conditioned tent, along with displays of helpful
information, including a list of "DOs" and
"DON'Ts" for visitors. Among the DON'Ts
were: "DON'T stop for long periods of time inside
of the Colossal Colon" and "DON'T horseplay
inside of the Colossal Colon." I thought the wisest
advice was: "DON'T leave your children
unattended."*

*If you're a parent, there are few
experiences more embarrassing than when you
report a missing child to the police, and the officer
asks you where you last saw little Tiffany, and you
have to answer: "She was entering a giant colon."*

*The Colossal Colon, shaped like huge
"C, " is made from plywood and polyurethane
foam. It has been sculpted and painted to look very
realistic, so much so that I was frankly reluctant to
crawl inside. I was worried about how far they
carried the realism. I mean, what if you got deep
inside there, and you suddenly were confronted, fun-
house-style, by some guy wearing a costume*

depicting an educational colon-dwelling character, such as Tommy Tapeworm, or, God forbid, Fred Food?

Fortunately, this did not happen. But the journey through the Colossal Colon is no walk in the park. You start out at the end labeled "Healthy Colon," and for a short while it's a pleasant enough crawl. But pretty soon you start running into bad things: first Crohn's disease, then diverticulosis, then polyps, then precancerous polyps, then colon cancer, then advanced colon cancer, and finally - just when you see the light at the end of the tunnel, and start to think you're safe - you find yourself face to face (so to speak) with one of mankind's worst nightmares: Hemorrhoids the size of regulation NFL footballs.

Shaken? You bet I was shaken. It was with weak knees that I emerged from the end of the colon (medical name: "The Geraldo"). There I was asked by a member of the Colossal Colon's entourage (yes, it has an entourage) to sign a pledge promising to consult with my doctor about my colon. I signed the pledge, although to be honest, I did not consult with my doctor. I consulted instead with my friend and longtime medical advisor Gene Weingarten, who is widely acknowledged to be the foremost hypochondriac practicing in America today.

Gene told me that he'd been screened for colon cancer, and that the procedure was not nearly as bad as I imagined. This is good, because I imagined that it involved a large, cruel medical technician named "Horst" and 70,000 feet of chairlift cable. But Gene assured me that it's nothing like that, and that they make you very comfortable (by which I mean "give you drugs"). Gene says they make you so comfortable that you'll be laughing and exchanging "high fives" with Horst (make sure he washes his hands first).

So I'm going to get the screening, darn it. I hope you do, too, assuming you actually get to see this column. I suspect some editors will decide not to print it, because it contains explicit words that some readers may find distasteful, such as "Geraldo." If you're one of those readers, I apologize if I offended you. But remember: I'm writing this because maybe - just maybe - it will save your life.

Ha ha! Not really. I'm writing this because I'm a humor columnist, and there was a giant colon in town.

But get yourself screened anyway.

©2003 Dave Barry

I put the paper down on my lap and wiped hysterical tears from my cheeks, partly from laughter and partly because Dave had done it. He had crawled through the Colossal Colon, written an entire column about his journey and then pledged to get himself screened. With one hilarious article, he had educated millions of people. His column was syndicated and published in newspapers across the country.

I realized that CoCo was doing *exactly* what she was supposed to do, and that I was definitely holding up my end of the bargain with Amanda. I folded the paper, closed my eyes and silently thanked Dave Barry.

The tour rolled on. We spent a week in Dallas, where my brother Rob came to visit CoCo, and another week in Houston. The farther into the tour we got, the more I realized how difficult it was to get people into the tent to talk about colorectal cancer. I had *almost* forgotten how embarrassed I was when I had symptoms and was first diagnosed. I had *almost* forgotten the X-ray tech who asked about my last bowel movement and the GI doctor with the crazy black snake lamp.

We spent two weeks in Chicago, first as guests of Roche at the annual meeting of the American Society of Clinical Oncology, where I was most amused at the prim and proper doctors who knelt by CoCo's hemorrhoids for photos. Then we were off to Pioneer Court for Chicago's public viewing of CoCo.

By the first afternoon, we'd already seen a few hundred people. Chicago looked promising. I was standing at the front of the tent, blowing up purple and green helium balloons, when a woman walked in and began to cry.

"Are you OK?" I asked, putting my hand on her arm.

"I'm sorry," she said. "This is just *a lot*. My brother is going in for surgery for stage IV colon cancer in an hour."

"I'm so sorry," I said and hugged her. "I'm a survivor, and you need to know that there is always hope." I handed her my business card. "If there is anything I can ever do, please don't hesitate to get in touch with me."

She thanked me and left the tent.

I was living out of my suitcase. I flew into a new city on Tuesday and arrived at the Colossal Colon early

Wednesday morning to speak at the press conference. We kept the doors open 11 hours a day, until seven p.m. on Saturday evenings, and then I'd fly home on Sunday morning. Between some cities we had a one-week break. For other cities, I would land Sunday night, do laundry and repack, and then start the cycle again on Tuesday. I loved it! And my new favorite thing was taking my seat on the plane and waiting for my seatmate to ask the inevitable.

"So, what do you do?"

I would look directly into the poor, unsuspecting eyes of my neighbor and say with a straight face: "I have a big colon and I travel around the country with it." The person next to me would raise their eyebrows, turn back to their book, magazine or computer and not say another word to me, or more often than not, tell me about their brother or mother or cousin or father who had been diagnosed with colon cancer. Statistics told me that colorectal cancer was the second leading cause of cancer deaths in the United States, but I was still shocked at how many people were affected by the disease.

We arrived in Phoenix in early June with our sights set on Los Angeles. It had been rumored that CoCo might make an appearance on *Jimmy Kimmel Live!*, and by the time I flew home from Arizona, it was no longer a rumor. CoCo and I were going to appear on the show.

When I landed at LAX, I got a voicemail from one of the show's producers. I called back as soon as I was behind the wheel of my rental car and found myself in a conversation that felt like an interview. At the end of our chat, he said he would call me back to let me know if I would be hosting the show that night.

Hosting? I thought I would be sitting on the couch answering questions. I could hardly contain my excitement. Forty-five minutes later, I got the call.

"Molly, you're going to be the host tonight," he said.

"You mean I passed my test?" I joked, trying to remain calm.

"Yes, and you're a natural," he said. "You have directions to the studio?"

"Yes."

"Good. I'll see you here at six p.m. We'll need you to cut some promo spots for us, and then we go live at nine p.m. here for the East Coast."

"Got it," I said. We hung up, and I sat in the car, stunned.

When I arrived at the studio in Hollywood, I felt completely out of my element. Everything was *so* Hollywood, and I was *so* upstate New York. The Cancer Research and Prevention Foundation asked me to wear my bright yellow Check Your Insides Out collared shirt, and I tried to make it look more hip with flare-leg jeans and some heels. It didn't work. Upon arrival, I was escorted directly to wardrobe for a new shirt.

Downstairs, in the makeup room, my hair was blown out and wax-like, camera-ready makeup applied. I put my new shirt on and felt a little bit more like I fit in. Then they sent me upstairs to cut some one-liners and promos that would run as the show went into and out of commercials.

After I was prettied up and my promos were done, I headed to the greenroom, which was much larger and had more of a party atmosphere than the one at the *Today* show. The lights were dimmed over velvet couches and there was an open bar, but I didn't dare have a drink. Instead, I paced and prayed that I would say the right things on live national television.

When it was time for the show to start, I was seated on a bar stool, on stage, with a microphone in front of me. I was next to the band and across the stage from Jimmy's desk, which was dark and empty. The theater was not. I really had to pee, but it was too late. The intro music started, and the crowd was on its feet. I stood up from my bar stool, pulled out my three-by-five cards and waited for my cue. The man behind the camera counted down on his fingers. Five. Four. Three. Two. Then he pointed at me.

"From Hollywood, it's *Jimmy Kimmel Live!*" With the music and the cheering crowd, I could barely hear myself as I yelled those words into the microphone. On a screen in front of me, I saw Jimmy, in a suit and tie, running down a street. Then he ran up a flight of stairs and into a building.

"Jimmy's guests tonight," I continued, "From *I'm with Busey*, Gary Busey and Adam de la Peña!" The crowd applauded loudly, and on the screen in front of me, Jimmy made his way up another flight of stairs.

"From AngryNakedPat.com, in our theater for the first time, it's Andy Milonakis!" Audience members whistled. "Music from The Donnas!" I screamed as Jimmy walked down a red-carpeted hallway. "And this week's co-host, Perry Ferrell!" The crowd continued to roar. I took a deep breath. "I'm your announcer, creator of the Colossal Colon, Molly McMaster. Now here's Jim-m-m-y Kim-m-m-el." My voice finally cracked as I yelled his name into the microphone over the crowd. Uncle Frank the security guard opened the main doors to the theater and Jimmy ran down the aisle and up the steps to the stage.

Once the crowd settled down, and I was safely back on my bar stool, Jimmy began his monologue.

"Thank you, everybody. Oh, we have a lot to get to. We have many, many, many things and let's start with the getting to my seat part ... Molly McMaster is here, and Molly, tell us what this is exactly."

"This is the Colossal Colon, for anybody who hasn't heard about it yet." I winked and the crowd cheered.

"... As you can see, it's a tremendous colon," Jimmy said, "a colon that is traveling across the country. Do people seem to like the colon?" Jimmy asked.

"People *lo-o-o-ve* the colon," I answered with drama in my voice. "We're actually headed to 20 cities. Los Angeles is city number 10. We're headed up the coast to San Francisco next week, and it's all put on by the Cancer Research and Prevention Foundation and Roche."

"Oh, good," Jimmy said. "There's a reason for this."

"Yeah, there's a big reason."

"Of the cities you've visited so far, which needs the most help with their colons, would you say?"

I put my thumb and forefinger to my chin and thought for a moment. "Possibly Miami," I said. "You didn't hear that from me though."

"Really?" Jimmy said. "I see. Now this is larger than the normal human colon, right?"

"Slightly," I said. "Would you like to hear a little bit of trivia?" I asked and went on without waiting. "If this were in – well," I stopped, realizing that the entire Colossal Colon wasn't on the stage. "This is a semi-colon, since it's not the entire Colossal Colon." The crowd laughed. "Work with me," I yelled to them.

"I guess I should have figured," Jimmy said. "If this colon were in a human, he'd be like the size of Shaq."

"Fifty to sixty feet tall," I corrected.

"That big? But this is only part of it?"

"This is a part of it. It's actually 40-feet long and four feet tall, and it's designed to teach people to check their insides out and get screened for colorectal cancer."

"Now how am I supposed to do that?" Jimmy asked.

"You go and get screened."

"Oh," Jimmy feigned an epiphany. "You go *to* somebody."

"When you turn 50, you get screened," I said, "unless you have family history, symptoms or risk factors. Then you should go sooner."

"I gotcha," Jimmy said.

"In truth, this is a serious subject, although it is funny, because that guy right over there is sitting in the hemorrhoids." I pointed at the cameraman preparing to film the first guest.

"Yeah, there's a guy in the colon," Jimmy said to fits of laughter. "And your goal is to get one of these on every playground in America, is that correct?"

"Absolutely," I said, pondering the possibilities.

"Was this your idea?" he asked.

"I'm 27 years old. I was diagnosed with colon cancer myself when I was 23, and my goal has been to raise awareness, especially in young people, because it can happen to anybody. It doesn't matter what color your skin is, or what language you speak, or what your dog's name is. It can happen to anybody."

"I got you. All right. Well, hey, when you do a breast awareness thing, come back with those," Jimmy said, and the crowd laughed and cheered again.

"You got it," I said.

"Thank you, Molly. So people, how do they get their colons checked? You're doing that after the show for people?"

"How do you get your *colons* checked?" I repeated. "We'll take you in the back room and you can bend over and we'll hook you up." The audience roared.

"It's going to be at Kenneth Hahn Hall, here in L.A. Wednesday through Saturday, and then in San Francisco – it's going to be popular in San Francisco," Jimmy said with a smile.

Jimmy and I bantered for another minute before the show cut to a commercial break. When the show returned, Jimmy's guests were forced to crawl through CoCo to get onto the stage for their interview. Gary Busey was less than eager.

I got back to my hotel room just in time to see myself announcing the show on the Pacific Coast delay and to hear Jimmy Kimmel talk about colon cancer on national TV. In my wildest dreams, I never would have imagined that this could happen.

CoCo officially opened in Los Angeles two days later, and Eric Davis, All-Star Major League Baseball player and colon cancer survivor, shared his story at our press conference. He was the first celebrity I had met who had been diagnosed with colon cancer and was willing to talk about it.

Sergei arrived in a convertible on Saturday afternoon, and as CoCo was packed up and loaded onto the truck, we headed up the Pacific Coast Highway to enjoy a three-day vacation. We sipped wine at a few vineyards, relaxed at Pismo Beach and stayed at the Post Ranch Inn in Big Sur, with its incredible views of the Pacific Ocean. Over dinner, we chatted about the Colossal Colon Tour and what would happen once I was back home. I didn't know what was next, but I knew that I was passionate about what I was doing. When we went back to our treehouse, a luxury room built on stilts and in a tree, nine feet off the ground, Sergei got down on one knee and asked me to be his wife. It was the most perfect night of my life.

Sergei flew home from San Francisco on the day the Colossal Colon opened. It was Gay Pride Week, and that celebration was happening in the same plaza as CoCo. As I flew home, I was still laughing at the man who had shown up in a crazy red jumpsuit with a boa and feathers in his hair asking if the colonoscope was available for parties.

I spent every flight reading and answering emails from survivors, patients, caregivers and CoCo fans from all over the country. On my red-eye flight home from San Francisco, I read an email from a woman in Chicago.

Dear Molly,

You probably won't even remember me, but I was the complete stranger in Chicago who came into the tent crying because my brother was going in for surgery. You came over and hugged me without question or judgment. I just wanted you to know that my brother's surgery was a success and he is doing very well.

Thank you so much for all that you are doing to raise awareness, and especially for being so kind to a stranger when she needed it most.

Best,
Beth

As the Colossal Colon crisscrossed the nation, life at home went on as usual, or at least it went on.

Just before CoCo arrived in Seattle Center, back in New York state, my 12-year-old nephew, Timmy, was diagnosed with Ewing's Sarcoma, a rare and aggressive form of cancer that normally strikes children or young adults.

"How can this possibly happen twice to the same family?" my sister-in-law, Aimee asked. I didn't have an answer. Aimee was pregnant with her third child but her first was beginning the battle of his life. Yet life went on, the same way it had when I was diagnosed.

A few weeks after Timmy's diagnosis, on July 21, 2003, Aimee gave birth to a beautiful baby girl named Jordan Katherine. I was elated about my niece, scared for my nephew, who had already started his chemotherapy and radiation treatments, and in awe of my sister-in-law, who kept putting one foot in front of the other.

As I touched down in St. Louis on a hot Tuesday night, there was a voicemail from my mother with more bad news. At my hotel, I called home from the balcony of my room, which overlooked the beautifully lit St. Louis Arch.

"Grandma had a stroke," Mom said.

"Is it bad?" I asked.

"We don't really know. She's in the hospital and isn't able to talk."

Grandma, who was 91, had moved from her condo in Ohio to upstate New York, where my parents could care for her. It was hard to imagine my grandmother, the matriarch, without a voice. She was not your typical sweet old lady.

I took a deep breath and remembered the day I was playing with my Breyer horses in her basement. I must have been five or six. "Molly?" she had called down from the kitchen in her sweetest grandmotherly voice. "Would you like a hot dog?"

"Yes, please," I had answered politely, just the way I'd been taught when respecting my elders.

"Well then, come on up here and I'll show you how to make it," she had barked back in a voice that I didn't know an old lady could produce. In my entire childhood up to that point, I'd never been as frightened of an adult as I was at that very moment, and just as suddenly as my grandmother had become crazed, I had lost my appetite.

I managed a small smile but realized that my eyes were brimming with tears.

"Mom, should I come home?" I asked, hiding my sadness.

"I don't know," she said. "I think that's up to you."

The next morning, I flew back to New York and drove directly to the hospital. I barely recognized Grandma. Her hair was disheveled, and she wore an ugly hospital nightgown instead of her usual matching skirt and blouse. Her false teeth sat in a cup next to her bed.

"I didn't even know she had false teeth," I said.

"Grandma always said that if you look better, people will treat you better," Aunt Lois said. That made sense. Grandma's hair was always carefully brushed, and her skirts were sharply pressed.

Sitting alone with her that afternoon, I held her frail little hand with the too-loose wedding ring that Grandpa had given her so many years before. I felt sorry for her, but couldn't shake a feeling of anger.

Growing up, I remember meeting my friends' grandmothers. I was jealous because they got hugs and kisses and unconditional love and praise. Just once, I wanted my own grandmother to tell me she loved me and that she was proud of me, but it never happened.

As I looked down at my Grandma, bedridden and speechless, I tried desperately to remember a time that she had actually told me she loved me, but I couldn't think of one. To me, it was a funny thing not being able to tell a person that you loved them. And over the past year or so, I had discovered not only that Grandma couldn't say it, but she also had an apparent discomfort with simply hearing the words "I love you," as if they were too honest or too improper. Of course, I took mischievous pleasure in this. When we said goodbye on the phone, I would say "I love you, Grandma," just to make her squirm.

"Uh, huh. You too," she had said back.

As I remembered this, I had tears in my eyes. But then I noticed that Grandma was looking intently at me from her hospital bed. I was still holding her hand. "I love you, Grandma," I whispered, and for the first time, I felt it in my heart.

She didn't have a voice, it was stolen by the stroke. But this time, I'm quite sure she mouthed the words, "I love you too."

I let out a breath, and with it, my anger disappeared.

Less than a week later, I watched Grandma take her last, peaceful breath in a bed set up in Mom and Dad's living room. She had never said she was proud of me and it took her until the end to tell me she loved me, but I finally understood her. Grandma was intelligent and serious and stern. Her family was her legacy. Proudly hiding her affection was her way of driving her seven grandchildren to be the best that we could be. She expected it, yet wanted us all to remain humble.

CoCo traveled through Detroit as we buried Grandma next to Grandpa in a cemetery in Delaware, Ohio. I rejoined the tour in Cleveland, where we were on the lawn of the Great Lakes Science Center, a few hundred yards from the Rock and Roll Hall of Fame. Every day, I looked at the steps where I had met Christian on my in-line skates three years before. It felt like a lifetime ago. I was such a different person then. Was he still in Cleveland or had he finally made it to Broadway?

Thousands of people had come through the exhibit since we had opened in Chapel Hill and many of them told us their stories of hope and tragedy. They told us that colonoscopies had saved their lives or that they were in treatment for colon cancer. People told us how they had lost family members and how family members had gotten life-saving colonoscopies. Story after story came through those doors, and my life went on. My nephew's cancer diagnosis, the treatments he was still enduring at age 13, and my grandmother's death, were still fresh wounds. After being on the road with CoCo for nearly nine months, I was finally hitting a wall of physical and mental exhaustion.

In Philadelphia, on our last day in Love Plaza, I needed to decompress and begged the staff not to call me for 30 minutes. I left the exhibit and ducked into a restaurant for a sandwich. Five minutes later, my phone rang.

"Yes?" I asked wearily, having already seen Hannah's number pop up.

"I know you told me you wanted a break, but there is a girl here that you *have* to meet."

"Han, c'mon," I whined.

"Molly, she drove three hours here just to meet you. She was diagnosed with stage IV colon cancer when she was 22."

I took a breath. "OK. I'll be right back."

I asked the waitress to wrap my sandwich and walked back to the tent where, standing next to Hannah, was a gorgeous young woman with long, dark hair.

She had colon cancer?

Erika told us that she was diagnosed in November of 2000, around the same time I was limping through the New York City Marathon. She was in college and engaged to be married but wasn't given much hope of survival. After three surgeries and one recurrence, she had been cancer-free for two years.

As the three of us stood around the Colossal Colon, Hannah and I told Erika about our goal to educate people, especially young people, in crazy ways. We told her we were starting a non-profit called The Colon Club, and that we wanted to be different from other organizations so we could grab the attention of young and old alike.

"We should do a calendar of young people all diagnosed under 50," Erika joked. "We can flash our scars at the camera!"

Her comment sparked my memory and a night in Colorado after hockey practice. I had been packing my hockey bag in the locker room when the rink attendant walked in to say hello.

"How was practice?" he asked.

"Good, thanks." I stood up from the metal bench and threw my bag over my shoulder. "What's that?" I asked, nodding at the magazine he had rolled up under his arm.

"Just Sports Illustrated," he said.

"*No way!*" I dropped my bag. "Is that the issue I've been hearing so much about? With Wayne Gretzky's wife?"

"Yeah," he laughed.

"Can I see it? I've heard it's awesome!"

"Sure," he said, handing me the magazine. I flipped through the pages until I found the photo of Janet Jones Gretzky, in a red bikini, leaned against a hockey stick. Her hair was in blond pigtails and she wore black hockey gloves, skates, white hockey socks and was somehow able to make the ugly hockey garter belt sexy.

"That is *awesome!*" I said again. "I want to have my picture taken like that someday."

"Molly," he snapped. "S*he's* a supermodel."

Back at the tent in Philadelphia, I flashed a mischievous smile at Erika. "A calendar is an *awesome* idea, and I already know what I'm going to wear!"

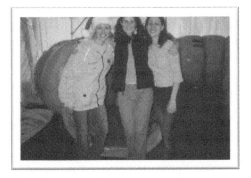

Me with Erika and Hannah

As I watched Erika walk away, I felt that I had found not a replacement for Amanda but another sister in the fight. I knew we needed to make her idea happen.

Finally, in late September, we reached our last stop, New York City. CoCo was set up in front of the Adam Clayton Powell Jr. State Office Building in Harlem. A giant colon seemed to be a tough gig there, but we had a strong showing. My brother, Rob, was in attendance for our final press conference. After Bo spoke, Dr. Mark Pochapin took the podium. He was the doctor for Katie Couric's husband, Jay Monahan, and she had picked him to head the Jay Monahan Center for Gastrointestinal Health, a clinical center of New York-Presbyterian Hospital and the Weill Medical Center of Cornell University. He talked about Jay's diagnosis and a book he had written titled *What Your Doctor May Not Tell You About Colorectal Cancer: New Tests, New Treatments, New Hope*. My story was in his book. I couldn't believe it.

As I went to the podium, I noticed that there was a class of nursing students in the back of the tent. When I told my story, I was thinking of them, hoping that they would never misdiagnose a young person with the same symptoms I had.

On November 1, 2003, the Colossal Colon Tour ended. I was relieved that things would finally slow down, but sad that it was over. I still couldn't believe that a silly little idea in the shower could become something that had, and would continue to have, an impact upon so many people. But I still had a promise to keep, and Erika's idea was getting me excited for our next big stunt.

23

AND THEN THERE WERE TWELVE

After decompressing at home for a few weeks, I began to grow restless. CoCo was booked to travel around the country for a second year, but this time she would visit private groups in smaller towns. I was scheduled to speak at a few of those venues but wouldn't be on the road nearly as much. It was time for something new.

In March of 2003, while CoCo was taking her first steps on the national tour, Hannah and I had filed paperwork to start a nonprofit called The Colon Club. Our mission was simple, but specific: to educate people, especially young people, about colorectal cancer in out-of-the-box ways. We knew that colorectal cancer organizations existed to provide education, support, research and advocacy. We wanted to do what no one else was doing. We wanted to educate in *crazy* ways, and young people were a virtually untargeted group. Our plan was to produce more wacky projects like CoCo, then work with established nonprofits to promote our projects within the colorectal cancer community. We would also use the media to get our message out to the general public.

In the spring of 2004, we brainstormed Erika's calendar idea. "It will be easy," we said. "We'll just get 12 survivors and take some pictures." We were in for an education.

To make a calendar, or Colondar, as we called it, the first thing we needed was funding. CoCo rentals brought in some money, but with the expense of moving her around, there wasn't enough left over to fund another big project. So we put together a serious proposal. The Colondar would be a 12-month wall calendar featuring survivors of colon and rectal cancer who had been diagnosed under the stereotypical age of 50. We sent our proposal to potential sponsors, believing it would be a no-brainer for someone to quickly put their name on it, a project that was sure to generate plenty of publicity. It didn't take long for one company to tell us they were interested, so we moved ahead on plans for the 2005 Colondar.

Hannah and I kept the project as economical as possible. Instead of renting a studio in New York City and putting our models up in ritzy hotels, I talked my parents into hosting models at their home on northern Lake George. Some of their neighbors agreed to host too. We would schedule the photo shoot on a long weekend in early summer. With our tight budget in mind, we asked friends and family to donate frequent flier miles, and we planned to do everything "in house," from booking flights and rides to and from the airport, right down to grocery shopping, cooking, making beds and cleaning toilets. Then, I contacted a local photographer.

"We are looking for three things with these pictures," I told Tom. "First, we want to be sure that our models' abdominal scars are visible."

"That will keep us locked into a handful of poses," he said. "That might be tough."

"I know," I said. "But I really think it's important to show that just because someone has colon cancer and a scar doesn't mean they can't still be healthy and beautiful."

"OK," Tom said. "What's the second thing?"

"We want jaws to drop," I said. "When people open the Colondar and realize that these beautiful models are just regular people with colorectal cancer, I want their chin to hit to floor!"

"But Molly, these are people with *no* modeling background, right?"

"Yes."

"It's going to be tough to get 12 strong photos with all amateurs."

How hard could it be to get 12 people to stand around and smile at the camera? "It'll be fine," I said.

"OK," Tom said, sounding unconvinced. "But make sure you have some beer and wine available for the models?"

"I'm on it," I laughed. I couldn't tell if he was kidding.

"What else?" he asked.

"Third, this is still about education, so we want to get the Colondar into the hands of people who wouldn't normally talk about colons."

"Is this a pin-up calendar?" he asked.

I hesitated. "Well, no."

"What are you planning for wardrobe?"

"Shorts, T-shirts, jeans."

"So, you want to sell your Colondars to the average Joe who knows nothing about colon cancer?"

"Yes."

"Sex sells," he said firmly.

"I don't want it to be trashy," I said.

"I understand. But colon cancer is pretty specific, and as you know, not something that most people like to talk openly about. If you want people who know nothing about colon cancer to buy your calendars, you have to give them a reason to buy them."

I bit my lower lip. I couldn't argue with that logic. "OK," I said.

Tom and I decided that our 12 models would wear bikinis, cut-off shirts, sports bras, shorts and miniskirts. We just needed to *find* those twelve models.

Over the next month, I called young survivors whom I had met or emailed. Erika, of course, was at the top of the list, and she wanted to pose as Miss November, her "cancer-versary" month. I claimed the title of Miss February, my birthday month and the anniversary of my own diagnosis. February would also match nicely with my red-bikini hockey theme. But we still needed 10 more models. I didn't even know 10 more young survivors, let alone 10 who would be willing to bare their bellies in front of a camera. We kept on searching.

Tammy, a twenty-something rectal cancer survivor who lived near St. Louis agreed to show her scar. In April, when I joined CoCo at an event in Nashville, I met a young survivor named Sara, who also joined the Colondar roster. She knew of a young survivor at her church and talked her into posing as well.

Before I knew it, 12 young strangers, connected by one disease, had agreed to meet in early June in a tiny hamlet in upstate New York and pose for some pictures. Flight arrangements were made, wardrobes selected, meals planned, photo sites scouted, and roommates set up.

A few weeks before the photo shoot, Hannah and I decided to send a few "test shots" to our sponsor, hoping to pass on our excitement. The sponsor's response stunned us. In an email, they said they could not put their name on something so "sexy." They were sorry, but they could no longer offer their financial support.

Crushed and discouraged, Hannah and I discussed our options.

"How can they pull out like that?" I asked, feeling defeated and trying to make sense of it. "This idea is awesome!"

"Amanda used to tell me that meeting you was one of the best things that happened to her after she was diagnosed," Hannah said.

"For me too," I said. "We understood each other in a way that someone who hasn't been through it couldn't possibly relate, and we didn't even have to talk about cancer."

"Then we have to do it anyway," Hannah said firmly. "We'll just have to figure it out as we go."

I knew she was right.

In less than 30 seconds we agreed that we *had* to go ahead with the project with or without our sponsor, because it really wasn't about the photos. There was no question that the Colondar was a terrific, out-of-the-box, awareness-raising idea, but the photo shoot would be about bringing 12 young survivors together. We hoped that they would form lifelong friendships and know that they were no longer alone, just like Amanda and me.

The strangers arrived in Albany, New York over the course of a few humid, late-June days in 2004. We picked them up at the airport, two or three at a time, in Sergei's SUV, driving the hour and 45 minutes to my parents' house on northern Lake George. We had 12 photos planned, with a mish-mash of themes, plus a cover. Based on our arrivals and departures, we had about 42 hours to pull it off.

We started Friday morning, with Sarah straddled over a triathlon bike wearing a funky athletic bikini. Far off in the scene was Rogers Rock, an historical landmark. But the clouds wouldn't cooperate. When our photographer finally accepted that Miss September would have a cloudy background, we got under way. Luckily, Sarah was a natural, and when her photo shoot wrapped up in less than an hour, the photographer and his two assistants packed up the set, loaded it into the car and drove to the next site, where they put it back together again for the next model.

We made it through three photos before breaking for a late lunch back at the house and asked the photographer to take a group shot of all the survivors together. I went through the house to round up the models, and as I made one last pass, I saw Mom on the front porch, staring down at the lawn where everyone was gathering.

"Mom?" I asked. "Are you OK?" She turned slowly and as her eyes caught mine, I saw her tears.

"They said you were the only one in the *country*," she said. "I never thought I'd see a day when there were 12 of you --- *together*."

I looked down at the beautiful young women and I really let it sink in. A knot began to form in my stomach as I swallowed the fact that our sisterhood was growing.

We continued shooting throughout the day and into the evening, and one by one, we knocked off a photo for each month. Most of the shots were taken in or around my parents' house and neighboring homes. Some were inside. Some were out, and on Friday night we even ventured out to a country bar. It was a rare gathering, a time when we could just be ourselves, survivors together, except for Linda. Her photo shoot was set up in the corner of the bar, with a band playing in the background.

On day two, we all caravanned south.

We started the day with Tammy crouched on a local school athletic field, holding a soccer ball. An hour or so later and a few miles to the south, Erika donned a black bikini and her fly-fishing gear and kneeled in the chilly Mettawee River, while Angie sat in a fold-up camping chair in a dirt parking lot off an old backcountry road. Samantha expertly styled Angie's hair with a curling iron plugged into the cigarette lighter in her car.

After Erika's photo shoot, everyone piled back into the cars and drove to the southern end of Lake George, where Angie posed in a navy-blue string bikini and in-line skates.

Then it was my turn. Samantha put my hair into pigtails and tied them with red bows. We went to a local ice rink and I went upstairs to change into a red bikini, covering it up with Dad's big red plaid flannel shirt, which hung down almost to my knees. I timidly went downstairs to the lobby, where I put on my hockey socks, garter, skates and gloves. My photo shoot would take place during a public skating session.

After the photographer's assistants set up their equipment, I picked up my hockey stick and nervously made my way out onto the ice, making a few small loops before getting settled into my place at the goal line.

Tom tested the light and had me try a few different poses. When he seemed satisfied, one of his assistants came over to take my flannel shirt. I hesitantly took it off, and as I handed it to him, I caught sight of a small crowd watching the show from the other side of the glass. My heart pounded hard against my chest. Even though I was wearing a bikini on an ice rink, I felt sweat on my back and hands. I looked wide-eyed at Tom, who crouched behind the camera and began snapping photos.

"Chin down a little bit," he said. "Eyes at me. Shoulders back." I followed each direction awkwardly while keeping the crowd in the corner of my eye.

Tom's head popped up from behind the camera. "Molly!" he snapped. "Eyes on me. Don't worry about them."

"OK," I said, closing my eyes and taking a deep breath. I opened my eyes and the camera clicked again.

"Show me a sexy smile," he said.

I laughed. My stinky hockey gloves and skates were hardly sexy.

Tom jumped out from behind the camera and approached me.

"Molly," he practically shouted, "Don't be the weak link here."

"Everyone's watching," I whined.

"Molly, *don't* be the weak link," he repeated. "This is *your* project."

I struggled through 45 minutes of camera snapping and posed as best I could until I was finally released. I snatched the flannel shirt and quickly put it back on.

As I stepped off the ice, my eyes met those of my seventh-grade health teacher and his daughter, who I had coached on the local 12 and under girls' hockey team. I was mortified.

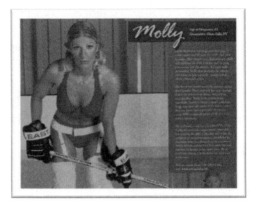

Miss February 2005

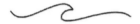

The photographer, his assistants, and some of the models began the hour-long drive back to the house. Our makeup artist hadn't been feeling well, so she had gone back earlier to lie down. We planned to resume shooting as soon as we all returned to the house.

Instead, when I got back and parked in the driveway, I caught my breath as soon as the car door slammed shut, realizing I had accidentally locked the keys *and the makeup* inside the car. I called Sergei, who was at least two and a half hours away, but would bring a spare key as soon as he could.

There was nothing I could do but wait. I headed to the dining room, where I heard talking and laughing. For the first time all weekend, the models and staff members were getting to know each. *Everyone* was relaxed and enjoying each other's company. I realized that locking the makeup in the car was not my best move, but it was exactly what we needed for a few short hours. We finally got the chance to talk about our lives, our diseases and the changes that had come since being diagnosed. It was what the entire weekend was *supposed* to be about. My father, normally so sarcastic and gruff, sat quietly at the back of the room taking it all in.

When Sergei arrived with the spare key, we got right back to work and finished our last photo around three a.m. Sunday morning in my parents' living room.

The weekend had been exhausting and exhilarating. On Sunday afternoon, after everyone had left and we were madly making beds and cleaning toilets, Tom pulled me aside.

"Molly, do you have a graphic designer to pull this all together?"

"No," I said. We still had no idea how we would pay to actually *print* the Colondar. We certainly didn't have money to hire a designer.

"You *have* to have a graphic designer," he said. "How were you planning to put the calendar together?"

"We hadn't really thought about that yet," I lied, not wanting to admit that I had made a silly little family calendar for Christmas a few years before and was preparing to take the photos to Staples and do it myself if need be.

"I know a guy that would be perfect for this project," Tom said. "His name is Troy Burns. He's an incredible designer. His father is dying of colon cancer." I got chills. "I'm going to give you his number, but you'll need to wait a few weeks before calling him."

When the weekend was over, we had put 1,500 miles on Sergei's SUV and were all running on next to no sleep. But we were onto something great. Even if the

Colondar itself flopped, we had brought 12 young survivors together. While the weekend wasn't perfect, our survivors knew that they were no longer alone. Now they all had one another, and there was no way to put a price tag on that. The rest was up to them.

A few weeks after the photo shoot, Tom let me know that Troy's father had lost his battle. It was time to call him.

"I've been looking for a way to get involved with the colon cancer cause," Troy told me. "I think this was meant to be."

Tom, Hannah and I selected the 12 photos and cover, and then passed them along to Troy, who tediously touched them up and tirelessly worked through the summer to design a calendar page for each model. I was in awe watching him work and couldn't believe we had thought we could do it all without a professional. On each page, he left room for a short biography, which I believed was the most important part.

The Colondar, with its beautiful young models baring gnarly abdominal scars, would attract attention but we couldn't miss the opportunity to educate about the disease. In the bios, which told a small piece of each person's story, we could tell people about symptoms, risk factors, surgical procedures, treatments, fertility and genetic disorders, among other things. Troy was a magician. Soon it was time to go to print.

The printer's quote for 10,000 Colondars was well over what we could afford. What little extra money we had was used on food and wardrobe for the models. We had no idea where we would find the money, but then Hannah's parents stepped in with an interest-free loan to

The Colon Club. It was a miracle, and in September of 2004, the first shipment of 2005 Colondars arrived on my doorstep. We were ready to raise awareness.

We approached a few other nonprofit organizations, thinking they would be thrilled to help promote the Colondar. Some were, but others acted as if we were their competition. So we turned our attention to the media. We wrote 12 separate press releases and sent them to radio stations, TV stations and newspapers in each of our models' hometowns. We also drew local attention, including in my hometown. Then we wrote a national release and sent it to everyone we could think of.

The 2005 Colondar was sold through our models and on The Colon Club's website, and right away we received emails from survivors and patients across the country. We heard from a woman in her mid-twenties who had recently undergone surgery for colon cancer. She wrote about how scary it all was. Her doctor told her that there weren't others like her. Now she was grateful to know that he was mistaken.

She told us that The Colondar was about self-esteem. It showed her that it was OK to bare her scar like a badge of honor, and she promised to wear hers proudly.

January came and went, and our media stories and Colondar sales slowed, but a second wave of attention came with the arrival of March, National Colorectal Cancer Awareness Month. The 2005 Colondar made the front cover of the New York Daily News in full color, with a three-page spread inside. I nearly fell over. That same day, an interesting email appeared in my inbox.

From: Christian
Sent: March 17, 2005
To: Molly
Subject: Hey...

... so I went and got the paper this morning...The New York Post and the New York Daily News and The New York Times. And I find you splashed all over.

I almost started to cry – perhaps it's a hazard of getting older, but when you look back and see where you've been and where you've gone and where you are, it's overwhelming.

I know more about your journey and your vision and your goals in the last few years than I know about most of the people I've met in the last 10 years of my life. I saw you this morning in the paper, and I just sat for a minute and smiled to myself – it's just beautiful. You look good, you sound good, you're strong, you are out there. It's just beautiful to see. It's a very powerful experience for me. Thank you. It's an amazing thing, life...isn't it?

Be good.
Christian

24

MAGIC DUST

T he feedback we received from the 2005 Colondar was overwhelming. Email after email arrived from survivors across the country who asked if they could share their story in the next Colondar. The project had to live on, so in October we created and sent out applications. Before we knew it, we had nearly 100 very worthy survivors asking to come to New York.

Believing that the more faces we could squeeze into the calendar, the more stories and angles we could showcase, we decided to double up on some of the pages for the 2006 Colondar, ultimately choosing 17 models, including five men.

As planning for the photo shoot began once again, we discussed minor changes. We talked about how we could make the weekend more about the people and less about the photos, to give our models more time to bond.

Our first decision was to have a barbeque on Saturday night.

We also found a new photographer, Mark McCarty. Troy had shown me some of his work online. He was a phenomenal photographer, with a passion for his work, but there was something else. When we met for dinner, and he told us that he had lost his first wife to breast cancer, I was certain he would bring compassion to our project. I told him that in the next Colondar, I wanted to be sure to show all of our models' abdominal scars, which ultimately hadn't happened in the first one.

"Model. Pose. Scar," Mark replied. He pursed his lips and looked up at the ceiling, apparently contemplating the challenge.

I bit my lower lip. Did he think I was crazy to put 17 strangers in front of a camera and expect magic?

"*OK*," he finally said, looking me straight in the eyes.

I knew that he was the perfect fit and would have the delicate touch our project needed.

After losing our one and only sponsor right before the photo shoot the year before, we were extremely lucky to still be able to pull it off. We knew we wouldn't get away with that again. This time, we decided to sell individual pages of the Colondar to sponsors, opening it up to different nonprofit organizations and businesses with a connection to colorectal cancer. Then we turned our attention to logistics.

The 2005 Colondar had us hopping until nearly three in the morning. We needed more time not just to shoot the photos but for the models to get to know each other. After discussing it with Mom and Dad and a few of the neighbors, we decided to add an extra day.

We also brought in an extra staff member to spread the workload. Flights would be booked so the models arrived and departed on the same days, eliminating multiple trips to the Albany airport.

Renting an RV was another logical solution to caravanning four or five cars from site to site and would give us a place to do hair and makeup out of the elements. It also allowed us to have food and drinks on hand, giving us the option of planning photo shoots that were farther away. The process was getting easier already, and our excitement was building once more.

Early June came quickly, and 17 survivors said hello on the dock at Mom and Dad's lakeside home.

On the set, Troy, Mark and Mark's two assistants were ready to go with the cameras and lights. Each model had their hair and makeup done in the RV and then walked over to the set, where Mark worked his magic behind the camera. It was fascinating to watch him bring out the very best in every single person. He made each one feel like the most gorgeous man or woman on earth and helped them overcome self-consciousness, lack of experience and a very emotional scar.

Behind the scenes, we found that renting the RV had not only simplified the preparations for the photo shoot, but it became another place where the survivors could bond. Each morning, I woke early and rounded up everyone scheduled for their photo that day, and each morning the same thing happened. The scheduled models would hop into the RV, and three or four others would follow, just because. For three full days, I drove them from site to site and just listened. They laughed and sang, shared secrets and tears, and bonded the same way Amanda and I had done. It was exactly what I had hoped for and it filled my heart.

On Saturday evening, the neighbors who opened their homes to the models joined us for dinner on the porch, where they could see for themselves what their generosity helped to create. Then, on Sunday morning, after the last model had left, we reflected on the weekend, thrilled to see that our subtle changes were allowing the photos to become secondary to the creation of a place where our survivors could meet *their Amanda*. Little did we know that it would only get better.

In the years since shooting the photos for the first Colondar back in the summer of 2004, a lot has changed. It truly has become so much more than "just getting 12 models and taking some pictures."

We've tried having 24 models, instead of 12, but nixed that after finding it to have taken away from the intimacy of the weekend.

We eventually turned Mom and Dad's garage into a studio, no longer having to worry about the weather, set-up, breakdown or drive time between photos that way, and there was absolutely no way anyone could lock the makeup in the car.

After ten years and a lot of growth, the photo shoot was moved to the Five Star Retreat, a private lodge outside of Nashville, Tennessee, where everyone would be able to stay under one roof. That same year, the Colondar was transformed into a full-color magazine called *On the Rise*, which referred to a study published in 2015 by the Journal of the American Medical Association (JAMA), showing a 51 percent increase in colorectal cancer incidence in adults younger than 55 years old between 1994 and 2014. Not only are the bios of each survivor longer and more detailed now, but more photos are included. *On the Rise* also contains articles that address other issues affecting young people diagnosed with colorectal cancer, like fertility, sex and dating with an ostomy.

Cell phones and Wi-Fi have dramatically changed the experience of the photo shoot, allowing the survivors to call, text or email home whenever the mood strikes them. It's so much different from the first few years, where everyone was present and we were assured that the models would connect with one another, since the only way to call home was to stand in line and wait your turn for the phone attached to the kitchen wall.

Social media has changed things too. The models who arrive at Colon Camp are now usually already Facebook, Twitter and Instagram friends, getting to know one another before the weekend and posting and tagging each other throughout.

But after all those changes through the years, and so many others, many things have still stayed the same. The process still starts with an application, which is reviewed by a committee that's looking to highlight different angles of the disease: genetic conditions, Irritable Bowel Disease, fertility issues, and patients who have done clinical trials. The committee also looks for people who were diagnosed early, people who were misdiagnosed, and long-term, late-stage survivors who show that there is *always* hope. Men and women of all stages, races and ages are considered, as long as they were diagnosed under age 50, since that's the stereotype we are still trying to break.

The survivors arrive from all over the country, not knowing what to expect, yet still ultimately finding it to be just like summer camp. They still talk, laugh, cry, swim, eat, stay up late into the night, and yes, even pose for photos. Then, sometime during the weekend, something magical happens, just like it did those first 10 years on Lake George. Troy calls it "magic dust," and says that it gets sprinkled over all of us. Whatever it is, there is no doubt that when the magic happens, it's life-changing.

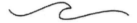

June 13, 2011

As someone who attended sleepaway camp, I knew what it was like to have camp end, and miss everyone so much that it hurt. You never knew when or if you would ever see them again.

This weekend, I attended my first Colondar shoot. A dozen younger colorectal cancer survivors descended upon a small burg on Lake George in New York. We arrived from all parts of the country, mostly not knowing one another, except from Facebook posts. But over the course of the four days, we shared the stories, created the memories and simply were ourselves. We didn't worry about how we looked, how often we needed the restroom, what our finances were or anything further than that weekend. We talked about oncologists, side effects, tumor staging, how we were first diagnosed and therapies.

I don't know exactly where I fit within the group. I was a young cancer survivor when I was in my twenties. Now I am the older cancer survivor in my forties, resigned to my situation and more concerned about my family. I'm the multiple cancer survivor with the genetic predisposition.

Some memories of the weekend will fade, but some will stick around. The smile on Belle's face as she laughed through the effects of chemo after traveling across the country. The frat boy's charm and wit of Adam as he joked his way through the weekend. Danielle's eyes and the way she absorbed everything as if through a video camera. Hugging Roger and kissing Todd's bald head as we listened to the bagpipes sing their lonesome song along the lake. The list of those departed.

On the Adirondack chairs, the signatures of those who have come before us. The "occupied" sign on the restroom that was always in use. The slushy machine churning out frozen alcohol all hours of the day. And the girls (sorry, my fatherly voice just took over). When I see them having cancer at such an early age, I could only think of my own children. Cathy's insistence that we live 50 years post-cancer like she has. Papa Jim drinking red wine with ice through a sippy cup. Refusing to let a day of rain keep us from climbing a mountain. Troy's creativity. I could go on.

The water and surrounding mountains of Lake George was a constant reminder that we are just sands in the hourglass of time. This truly wasn't about the photography, although the camera staff made me feel special and look even better. However, the photo shoot was my snapshot in time. I haven't felt this good in years, and since I don't know the duration of my future, I, like most with me this weekend, want this to be how I am remembered.

My life goes on. And for the first time in a very long time, I slept through the night.

David Dubin
Mr. January
2012 Colondar

25

CROSS-CHECKING COLON CANCER

During the summer of 2005, while Troy was hard at work putting the 2006 Colondar together, I was swinging a golf club at the local country club. I didn't *love* golf, but the Adirondack Frostbite, the local UHL team formerly known as the Adirondack IceHawks, was holding a tournament to benefit The Colon Club. Suddenly, I was a golfer.

After a less than stellar round, I returned to the clubhouse where the team's new owners, Barry Melrose and Steve Levy, both of ESPN, mingled with the crowd, along with many of the Frostbite players and the newly hired head coach, ex-NHL player Marc Potvin.

"So, Barry," I asked. "Have you had your colonoscopy yet?"

"I'm not getting that thing," he said.

"Oh, c'mon," I teased. "It's not so bad."

"Hey, we just met," he said. "Let me warm up to you first?"

"Fine," I laughed, "but I'm going to keep after you."

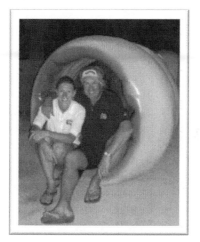

Me & Barry Melrose with CoCo

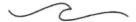

Despite my lack of golfing experience, the day had been fun, but the real surprise came when Coach Potvin offered me a job with the Frostbite.

"I already have a job talking about colons," I joked, assuming he was kidding.

"It can be part time," he said. "Think about it. We'll talk next week."

Working with a professional hockey team would definitely be fun, and a nice break from colons, I reasoned. Before the week was out, I had accepted the coach's offer to become the players' "handler." I would spend a few hours each week escorting players to schools, libraries, youth hockey practices and lunches with local seniors. It *really* was a nice break from cancer, but it wouldn't take long for my two worlds to collide.

One afternoon in late fall, while walking through the arena with Coach Potvin, he looked at me and nodded at the ice.

"Molly, we should suit you up to play with the guys some night."

"Very funny," I said.

"Seriously," he said, stopping in front of his office door. "We can tie it into your colon cause. Convince the UHL commissioner, and let's do it."

A meeting with the commissioner of the United Hockey League was set, and the next time he was in town for a game, I met with him in the front office during intermission. I was armed with a stack of thick binders filled with magazine articles and newspaper clippings from the past six years of raising awareness, as well as a few photographs and a video of me skating. I wanted to show him not only that I had experience attracting the media, but that I could also hold my own on the ice.

"I'm a cancer survivor myself, so I know where you're coming from," he began after I had given my best pitch. My heart sunk and I prepared myself to hear that it was too dangerous and that a woman had no business being on the ice with those boys. "I think it's a *great* idea, and while you're at it, I think you should travel to all 14 of the UHL teams and play a shift with each one during the month of March. Let's get you some awareness of colon cancer and your Colon Club."

I left the Frostbite office in shock, trying desperately not to scream with joy. Knowing there weren't many private places in the arena during a game, I followed the underground passageways to the opposite end of the building, where I knew spectators didn't usually go. I hid in one of the pits and dialed Rocky.

"Rock! I just spoke with the UHL Commissioner! He's going to let me play a shift with every team in the UHL during the month of March to raise awareness of colon cancer!"

"*What?* Do you mean to tell me that I spent months traveling around the country trying out for teams and getting cut, and you're going to play for every team in the league? Are you *kidding me?*"

As he said the words, I realized that my dream of playing for the U.S. Women's Olympic team would never happen, but this was definitely a close second.

After I hung up with Rocky, I took a breath. Calling him with that kind of news was easy. Calling Sergei to tell him that I would spend a month on the road playing hockey with a bunch of men? Not so much. He always supported my crazy ideas, but this one might be over the top. I dialed nervously.

"Hello?" he answered. "How did your meeting go?"

It was six years since we'd met on the ice for the first time, but I never tired of that Russian accent.

"Um," I stalled. "Better than I expected."

"They're going to let you play?"

"Sort of."

"What do you mean?" he asked. "That's great!"

"The commissioner actually suggested that I play for all 14 teams in the UHL throughout the month of

March." I paused, waiting for his reaction and hiding my excitement.

"Baby, that's *awesome!*" he said.

Once again it was going to take a miracle to find funding. Hannah and I threw together another sponsorship proposal and sent it to Fleet Pharmaceuticals, which quickly agreed to sponsor the *entire* tour. Eneman, Fleet's walking enema mascot, was our miracle and my new best friend. He would join me in all 14 cities, handing out stuffed Eneman dolls while working the crowds and posing for pictures.

Although Eneman would be the perfect partner to draw more attention to colon cancer, we knew that people weren't going to rush out and get a colonoscopy just because they saw him walking around the arena, or me on the ice. We wanted to pack as much awareness as possible into "The UHL Cross-Checks Colon Cancer," and while we had some great ideas, our brochure had me worried. I didn't want to spend a lot of money on boring clinical-type pamphlets and then find them on the floors and in the trash. I wanted people to actually take them home and *really* read them. But what would people actually pick up and keep? Something pocket-sized, and the less wordy the better. How about my Colondar photo? That was pure Colon Club craziness. We decided to create a Limited-Edition Molly McMaster UHL hockey trading card. Sure, the picture was a little racy, but people would definitely pick it up and look at it. It would also draw hockey fans to the education tables that we would have in each arena. At the tables, I could tell my story, answer questions, talk to other survivors and maybe even autograph a hockey card or two.

Unfortunately, not all the UHL teams were thrilled with the revealing picture of me in my red bikini and pigtails, so we had a second made in which I wore my real hockey uniform and an official UHL jersey.

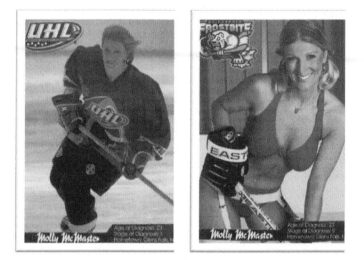

Limited Edition Molly McMaster Hockey Cards

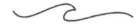

We printed both cards with each team's logo on the front. Underneath the photo it said:

Molly McMaster
Age at Diagnosis: 23
Stage at Diagnosis: II
Hometown: Glens Falls, N.Y.

On the back of the card, instead of my hockey stats, we listed the symptoms, risk factors and information about colorectal cancer. It was pocket-sized, short and sweet. It was *brilliant.*

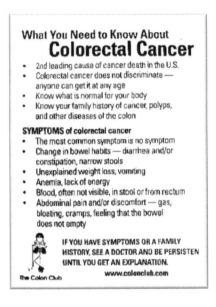

Hockey Card Back

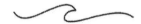

While Hannah and I continued to run The Colon Club, I began lifting weights with a trainer and continued to play hockey with my women's team. I also joined the Frostbite for practice a few times a week.

On February 19, 2006, I celebrated my 30th birthday and my seventh-year cancer-free. One week later, I stepped onto the ice in Lake Placid, my lucky necklace around my neck, for my third Empire State Winter Games. I left the ice as a gold medal winning defenseman, but even that thrill was not the highlight of the weekend. Later that same day, I would skate onto another sheet of ice as the first-ever female Adirondack Frostbite player in the United Hockey League.

With my heart in my throat, I got dressed in a small locker room down the hall from the Frostbite and prepared for my first UHL appearance against the Richmond Riverdogs. There was a knock at the door.

"Come in," I answered.

"Hey!" My eyes nearly popped from my skull as I recognized the RiverDogs very large and very intimidating enforcer immediately. "You know that you and I are dropping the gloves at center ice the second the puck drops, right?" He winked, allowing me to loosen up slightly.

"Sure we are," I said with a smirk but prayed he was kidding.

After the warm-up, I joined the team in the locker room for my first UHL pre-game speech. The boys were silent while the coach walked them through the game plan, and I didn't dare say a word, but as I sat with shaking knees, one of my teammates handed me a cup of Gatorade and smiled.

"Cheers," he said. We tapped our Dixie cups together and he gave me a wink.

At four minutes to game time, I stood with the rest of the team and walked to the tunnel. "Good luck," my teammate Rapper said, flashing a calming smile. I closed my eyes.

The announcer began calling the starting lineup, while AC/DC's "Thunderstruck" blared throughout the arena. The captains slapped our shin pads with the blades of their sticks as we walked by. But my knees were still shaking.

"Starting at center," the announcer shouted, "Hugo Belanger!" Hugo sprinted onto the ice to a cheering crowd while I listened to my heart pound in my ears.

"And finally, appearing for the first time with the Adirondack Frostbite tonight," the announcer yelled, "on left wing, Molly-y-y-y-y McMaster-r-r-r-r!" I took a breath, swallowed hard and opened my eyes, then bounded into the darkened arena while the spotlight chased me. Finally, I smiled, and I couldn't peel it from face.

We skated around our end of the ice for a few moments before the teams headed to their respective benches, and I lined up on the blue line with the rest of the starting players for the national anthem. We faced the flag with our helmets at our sides, and as the music began, I closed my eyes, imagining myself as a starting player for the U.S. Women's Olympic team. I opened my eyes and glanced at Hugo on my right and Rapper on my left. I looked to my bench, where all of my Frostbite teammates were wearing the Blue Star patch on their jerseys, a symbol representing the fight against colon cancer. *Every* player on *every* team in the UHL would wear that patch on their home jersey throughout the month to raise awareness of colorectal cancer. Then I looked up at the crowd. Eneman's pointy orange head bobbed up and down among the fans at the top of the arena, and as I perused the crowd, even from center ice I could see people holding something pocket-sized in their hands. I smiled. As the anthem continued, I looked back at the American flag and felt a wave of pride. I had never been asked to an Olympic tryout, but I was doing something just as awesome. Maybe I would even save some lives with this little hockey tour, and for me, that was better than any Olympic medal.

Just before the game began, a red carpet was rolled onto the ice, and a group of colorectal cancer survivors walked out with Eneman to meet the two team captains at center ice for the ceremonial puck drop. I watched with a smile, thinking back to Rolling to Recovery Night with the Adirondack IceHawks. That night, when I stood over the puck, I thought that face-off would be the closest I would ever get to my dream. Yet here I was six years later, *playing* in the UHL on that very same ice.

Tonight, the survivors held an official UHL Cross-Checks Colon Cancer puck with the special logo: a blond pig-tailed stick figure with pink hockey gloves and a squiggly colon. The little logo was just one more way to make people talk.

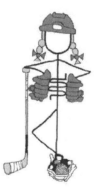

The UHL Cross-Checks Colon Cancer Logo

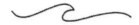

At center ice, the group dropped the puck for the captains, and with his stick, Hugo gently pulled it back to himself, picked it up and handed it to one of the survivors. Then the ref blew his whistle and I followed the starters to center ice for the opening face-off, lining up on left wing across from a Roanoke player who wasn't much bigger than me. I let out a breath of relief.

The referee looked from one goalie to the other and then to the scorekeeper. Then he dropped the puck. Immediately I found myself following the play into our own defensive end, and as suddenly as it had begun, my anticlimactic first shift in the UHL was over in just under 30 seconds. I skated back to the bench to hear the announcer speaking over the crowd. "Ladies and gentlemen, colorectal cancer is the second leading cause of cancer death in the United States, but one of the only forms of cancer you can test for and remove before it starts." This was one of dozens of facts about colorectal cancer that would be announced over and over in each arena all month long.

When the horn sounded to end the first period, I retreated back to my small locker room for a shower while Polyp Man danced around the ice on skates to "I Feel Like a Polyp," and the crowd tossed beach balls emblazoned with more facts about colorectal cancer.

"Oh, educate we will," I laughed, singing along to the tune of Shania Twain's "I Feel Like a Woman." Who in the crowd would have a beach ball when the music stopped? In a few minutes, I would meet those people at the table on the concourse and give them each an official UHL Cross-Checks Colon Cancer puck.

As the horn sounded to start the second period, I wound up an interview with an Associated Press reporter and then made my way upstairs to the education table. I was shocked to see a long line of autograph seekers, all of them holding Limited Edition Molly McMaster hockey cards. I couldn't help but laugh … and blush.

Somewhere in the middle of the line was Kim Troisi-Paton, a stage III colon cancer survivor and local resident who would soon become a 2007 Colondar model. Before Kim succumbed to colon cancer in August of 2007, The Colon Club would help her create Posterior Designs: Cards for Any Colon Occasion – funny and sometimes crass greeting cards that asked recipients to get their colonoscopies and thanked others who already had. She would also start Cut the Cheese to Cut out Colorectal Cancer, a fundraiser that would eventually support the Kimberly Fund, whose mission would be to help children who lost a parent or caregiver to colon cancer.

At the end of the night, I took my game jersey down to the Frostbite locker room and had every player on the team autograph it. I would do the same thing with each of my game jerseys. At the end of the month we would auction them off to raise money for The Colon Club.

The weekend was a whirlwind, but there was no time to rest and I wasn't complaining. It was the beginning of what would turn out to be a long, exhausting and *awesome* month.

Three days later, Sergei dropped me off at the back entrance to the Danbury Ice Arena in Connecticut just in time to suit up for morning practice with the Trashers. I was grateful to have the opportunity to practice with them, and I think they were impressed, or at least relieved to know that I could stay on my feet. What surprised me the most though, was how the Frostbite's biggest rivals welcomed me. Even the coaches took me under their wings.

"Hey," one of my teammates said as we left the ice. "My grandmother died of colon cancer. This is awesome, what you're doing."

That night, as I stood in the pit with the team, waiting for the starting lineup to be called and for my second shift in the UHL, my heart raced, but this time my knees weren't shaking. I felt a nudge and looked up at my towering teammate.

"Hear that?" he said. Music was screaming through the arena, but I hadn't noticed it. This time, the starting lineup would skate out in the darkened arena with the spotlight shining down and the smoke machine spitting to Aerosmith's "Dude (Looks Like a Lady)."

"Please welcome to the Trashers starting lineup tonight," the announcer shouted over the crowd, "Molly-y-y-y McMaster-r-r-r!" It would never get old.

I leapt out onto the ice through the smoke, just as Motley Crew began shrieking "Girls, Girls, Girls."

After the anthem had been sung, the two captains lined up at center ice with Eneman for the ceremonial puck drop that would honor survivors in almost every arena. In Danbury, two more 2007 Colondar models were there to do the honors.

The Muskegon Fury player across the red line winked at me as we faced off, and the referee dropped the puck. My centerman quickly won the faceoff, drawing the puck back to his defenseman, who held it for a few moments and then passed it across to the other Trashers defenseman. I raced toward our offensive end, curling toward center ice. Suddenly, the puck slapped my stick and I took a few strides before making a long pass to my opposite winger, who skated in and took a shot on net before the goalie gloved it and the referee blew his whistle to end my shift. I looked up at the clock. Nearly a minute had passed.

Muskegon won the game, and that night Sergei drove the three hours home while I slept in the passenger's seat. I was exhausted already, but there was no time to rest during this dream come true. The next morning, I flew to Michigan, where the Flint Generals welcomed me with shaving cream in my glove. I loved it. The gag was part of the hockey camaraderie I had always longed for.

The next evening I found myself in the Motor City Mechanics locker room, just outside of Detroit. The first time I got onto the ice with each team was like another tryout, so I welcomed the morning practices, but the Mechanics had come in late from a road trip the night before, which meant no morning practice. My first introduction with them would be in the locker room just before the game.

As I walked in, the coach pointed to an empty locker. The player sitting next to it, who had a strange likeness to Wayne Gretzky, cleared a few of his things from the seat. I nervously walked across the room, past 20 young, male players, and the coach spoke up.

"Guys, this is Molly. She's the girl that will be skating with us tonight."

As quickly as the coach said it, Wayne Gretzky's look-alike began putting everything back down on the bench. I was confused.

"Your seat," he said, pointing grandly to his lap. I learned long ago that men's hockey was a kill-or-be-killed space.

"I'm not sitting there," I quickly snapped. "I don't know where that thing's been!" The room erupted in laughter and cheers, and I sat down next to him smiling.

"I'm Brent," he said, putting his hand out for me to shake. "Gretzky."

The Motor City Mechanics were the biggest guys in the UHL, most of them well over six feet tall. To me, that translated into the most intimidating team. Still, when I stepped out onto the ice for the pregame warmup, I was calm. Five minutes in, one of my teammates came up behind me in the drill line.

"Where'd you play college?" he asked.

"I didn't."

"*Seriously?*"

One point, McMaster.

After the starting lineup had been called and the national anthem sung, I took my spot at left wing as my centerman lined up to take the face off. I watched, my mouth agape, as he batted his opponent's stick and said something to the referee. Before I knew what was happening, the referee was directing him out of the faceoff circle and waving me in. My heart pounded in my ears. I had been playing defense ever since my first year playing hockey when I couldn't figure out the offside rule, so my coach decided it was just easier to put me in the back. I had practiced face-offs a few times over the years, but nothing serious, yet there I was about to take the draw in the United Hockey League against a guy that was easily six inches taller than me.

Before I could even start an argument, I found myself bent over the face-off dot watching the puck in the referee's hand and hearing Rocky's voice in my head.

"On the face-off, you *never* take your eyes off the puck," Rocky said, "and as soon as that ref starts moving his hand like he's going to drop it, start swinging."

The ref turned to one goalie, then the other. Then he turned to the scorekeeper and back to us, but I never took my eyes off that puck. I watched his knuckles whiten just slightly. Then his elbow rose, and he released. The puck fell to the ice in slow motion, and I quickly began sweeping my stick front to back, just like Rocky told me. How it happened, I'll never know, but I pulled the puck back through my skates to my defenseman, and suddenly we were skating hard into our offensive end. The puck flew around the boards and out of the zone.

I looked to the bench, preparing to end my shift as a Motor City Mechanic, but before I could even change direction, the puck was headed back toward the opposing goalie. I raced across the blue line and directly to the net, parking myself in front of the goalie and feeling the shoves of a very large Roanoke defenseman. Then, there it was. The puck was inches from my feet, sitting in the goal crease. The goalie was down on his knees at the other side of the net, leaving me alone to score. I batted my stick at the resting puck, but I couldn't move. The six-foot-plus Viper defenseman was the only thing standing between me and the title of "First Female to Score in a Professional Men's Hockey Game," but I couldn't fight through him. I struggled until the goalie finally snatched up the puck and the referee blew his whistle. My moment was over. I had *almost* scored. *Almost.*

After the whistle, I headed back to the bench amid a team filled with excitement.

"You were *so* close!" one said, tapping the top of my helmet.

"That was *awesome!*" another chimed in.

The next morning, I drove to Port Huron. No practice that morning meant another pregame warmup tryout for me, so I went to the rink to get acquainted with the team before the five o'clock game.

A vase of flowers awaited me in my locker room, and I chuckled at the thought of flowers for a hockey player. I dressed for warm-ups and joined the team in the locker room where my new teammates quickly caught sight of the black, metal full-face cage on my helmet.

"Yo, Bird Cage," one of them said to me with a smirk.

"Make fun if you will," I said, "but I still have all my teeth."

Before we headed out to the ice, the coach asked me to take the ceremonial puck drop. I skated to the red carpet where I met Eneman with an older gentleman who held a squiggly colon-girl puck. I shook his hand.

"Thank you for what you're doing," he said, and we gave each other a knowing smile. Then I bent over the ice with a Muskegon Fury player to take my first ceremonial faceoff.

The older man dropped the puck and I quickly began swinging my stick at it, just like Rocky had taught me, pulling the puck back between my feet. It slid 30 or so feet before coming to a stop somewhere in the middle of the ice.

"Ha ha!" I bragged to the Fury player, but he only looked at me with bewilderment.

"Hey, McMaster," he said. "*Ceremonial* puck drop. You know you're just supposed to pull the puck back and then hand it to the person who dropped it, right?" I instantly turned bright red. "Nice one," he said laughing and shook my hand. "I'll see you in Muskegon." He skated back to his bench, leaving me red-faced.

Before I could slink away, one of the Flags' owners handed me a plaque and announced into the microphone, "The Port Huron Flags would like to welcome Molly McMaster to Port Huron and present her with this plaque commemorating the first woman to play in a UHL game in Port Huron, Michigan on this day, March 5, 2006 versus the Muskegon Fury."

"Hey, Bird Cage," one of my teammates yelled when I got back to my own bench. "Nice faceoff!" They all laughed while I quietly returned to red.

At the opening faceoff, the Fury winger on the other side of the blue line hooked his stick around my waist, but I broke free when the puck dropped and stuck my tongue out at him before skating away. It was only my second meeting with the Fury, but they were quickly becoming my favorite team.

Muskegon won the game again, and I flew home to spend 24 hours with Sergei and do some laundry before driving four hours to Elmira, New York, on the next day.

Just like in 2003, my year traveling with the Colossal Colon Tour, I was living out of my suitcase. The schedule was hard, booked solid with travel, practices and games. I finally understood why many of the Frostbite players always told me they were going home for a nap after practice. The lifestyle was exhausting and there seemed to be little time for anything else. Then came Elmira, in the Southern Tier region of New York state.

A few weeks before I met with the UHL commissioner, I received an email from a group in the Southern Tier asking if we could partner in March for a big project. When I confirmed with them, they were thrilled and said that they would line up some speaking engagements and radio and TV interviews while I was in town.

I arrived in Elmira and went directly to the arena to tape a radio interview that would air later that day. Then I woke up early the next morning, game day, for a second radio interview, before driving to a local hospital to tell my story over breakfast to a group of doctors and nurses.

Then it was back to the arena for practice. We went through a few drills, and while standing in line awaiting my turn, one of the players nudged me. His face wore a serious expression.

"My Dad had colon cancer," he said. "Thanks for doing all this."

"Are you kidding?" I said. "I get to put the two things I love together – hockey and colons." I was having so much fun I almost forgot it was for a cause.

After practice, I left my gear in my locker room and went to a second hospital to tell my story to doctors and nurses again, this time over lunch.

At the arena that night, I did another interview, this time with the game's radio caller. Throughout the game, he would announce the same list of colorectal cancer facts that we had given to the arena announcer, just like all the other teams were doing, and then the interview would play during the second intermission. We weren't just educating the fans in the building, but also the ones who had missed the game that night.

"How has your experience in the UHL been so far?" he asked.

"I'm exhausted and running on adrenaline," I admitted, "but this is the opportunity of a lifetime. I'm playing professional hockey! Who gets to do that? And then on top of it, we are raising awareness of colorectal cancer, a disease that no one wants to talk about it. Here in Elmira, the awareness is through the roof! It's awesome!"

"What about the players?" he asked. "How are they reacting to you?"

"This morning during practice, one of the guys told me that his father had colon cancer and he actually thanked *me* for what I was doing. I'm the one that should be thanking *them*!"

When we finished, I went to my locker room to find my jersey on a hanger and my pants and socks hanging from a hook. My skates had been sharpened and sat neatly on the floor, and my shoulder, elbow and shin pads were lined up next to my seat. I sat down and took a deep breath, taking it all in. One by one, the teams were taking me under their wings, treating me like one of their own and then thanking *me* for doing what I was doing. The whole experience was simply mind blowing.

That night after my shift, Elmira tanked the game, losing to the Rockford IceHogs 10-2, but Elmira had been the biggest success so far, reaching far beyond the walls of the arena.

Early the next morning, I boarded a plane in Elmira on what would become a very long day. When I landed in Chicago a few hours later, my troubles began when my flight to Muskegon was canceled.

"I already have you booked on the next flight," the airline employee said, while typing away.

"When is that?" I asked, assuming I would arrive in Muskegon at midnight.

"One p.m. tomorrow," she said. Panic tore through me as I did the math.

"Um," I started. "That won't work."

"I'm sorry, Ma'am, but that's the only flight we have."

My mind raced. Practice with the Fury was at 10 a.m. I wouldn't make that, but I still needed to be at the rink by five for the game. If tomorrow's flight was late or canceled, I could miss it altogether. What could I do? I looked around and a Hertz sign caught my attention. I turned back to the woman.

"How far is it from here to Muskegon?" I asked.

"I'd say about 250 miles," she said.

"How long will it take to pull my bags?" I asked.

"I don't think we can do that," she said.

"I need to be on the ice in Muskegon tomorrow morning at 10 a.m.," I said, knowing she had no clue what I meant, "and I need my hockey bag and sticks off that plane. *Please!*" I pleaded.

She picked up the phone and made a call.

"It could take up to three hours," she said, hanging up.

"Thank you so much!" I said. Then I looked back up at the Hertz sign and followed the arrows.

After I had secured a car, I found my way back to baggage claim and waited. Two and a half hours later, my oversized hockey bag appeared on the belt, followed by my suitcase and then my navy-blue stick bag with the colon cancer star on it. I grabbed them all and dashed to the exit. I wanted to be in Muskegon before midnight.

As I waited at the curb for the shuttle, I overheard two young women discussing their options after their own canceled flight.

"Weren't you just on my flight?" I asked, recognizing one of them.

"Yes," they said in unison.

"The airline didn't give us a hotel voucher," one of them said, "and we don't have enough money to stay anywhere." I looked them over for a few seconds.

"I have to be in Muskegon by tomorrow morning," I said, "so I rented a car. Do you want a ride?" They looked at each other and then back at me. "I'm not a weirdo, I promise!" I laughed.

"*Really?*" one of them asked. "Thank you so much! We would *love* a ride home!"

We left Chicago at rush hour, and the first thing I learned as we pulled away from the airport was that one of the women was a nursing student.

"I didn't know someone could get colon cancer so young," she said. There wasn't a moment of awkward silence during the entire five-hour trip, as I told them my story and why I was going to Muskegon, and they told me about their families and school.

"I'll have a set of tickets at the will-call window for you tomorrow night," I said when I finally dropped them off. "Thanks for riding with me. I'm kinda glad our flight was canceled."

I got to my hotel in Muskegon just after 10 p.m. Exhausted, I went right to bed.

When I arrived at the L.C. Walker Arena the next morning for practice, the equipment manager handed me a white helmet to match the rest of the team, before closing the door to my private locker room. I sat on my bench and looked it over. The UHL only required a half shield, but I didn't want to get a puck or stick in the face, so I normally had a full, black metal face cage that had gotten me the nickname "Birdcage" in Port Huron. My new helmet, called a "bubble," had a clear plastic face shield to protect my eyes and a plastic cage at the bottom to protect my smile.

I suited up for practice and when I heard the team making their way out to the ice, I pulled my new helmet on, opened my locker room door and followed them.

"Hey," I heard behind me as I stepped onto the ice. I turned to see another Fury player wearing a face shield just like mine. He tapped his stick on the clear plastic in front of my eyes. "My bubble's better than your bubble," he bragged before skating off.

"Don't listen to him," the player next to me said. "He's just mad because he got his nose broken and isn't allowed to wear a half shield until the doctor clears him." I laughed. "You can make fun of him too. By the way, our record is awesome when you're in the building, but it's good to finally have you at our end of the ice."

I didn't know whether to be flattered or mad.

That night, I couldn't get off the ice fast enough after my most terrifying UHL shift to date. The Kalamazoo Wings wasted no time, quickly winning the faceoff and rushing into our end, before ringing the puck off the post. Thankfully they didn't score, and my plus/minus remained at zero.

After the first period, I showered, dressed and walked upstairs to find our education table on the main concourse. Once again, I was met by a long line of autograph seekers holding hockey cards. The girls who had driven up from Chicago with me the day before greeted me, and a group of gastroenterology nurses proudly showed off their homemade Eneman baseball caps with large, pointed orange cones on the tops and matching earrings.

After nearly an hour, the line finally began to thin and an adorable young woman who looked to be in her late teens shyly approached me.

"Are you enjoying the game?" I asked.

"I was diagnosed with colon cancer when I was 13," she said quietly, handing me a hockey card to autograph. I was startled. She was practically a baby.

"What's your name?" I asked.

"Marcy. I never knew there was anyone else so young out there like me," she said.

"You've never met another young survivor?" I asked.

"Never," she said. "My doctor said it was impossible."

"I know the feeling," I said. "How would you feel about posing in a calendar of survivors? We have an amazing weekend and you can meet other 'youngsters.'"

"Seriously?" she said, beaming. "I'd love that."

I wrote my phone number and email address on a scrap of paper and hugged her. As she walked away, I prayed that I would hear from her.

That night, the Fury won the game, and the team began calling me their good luck charm.

The next morning, after making the hour and a half drive to Wings Stadium in Kalamazoo, Michigan, I met the coach in his office before practice. He wasn't a very big guy and wore glasses that made him look too smart to be a hockey player.

"I need you to sign your contract," he said, handing it to me. I looked it over and laughed.

"I'm getting paid 'for the love of the game,' huh?" I asked.

"That's correct," he said smiling. "You know the UHL isn't made of money."

"I'm good with that."

The Port Huron Flags were in town that night and they teased me and slapped their sticks against my shin pads as we passed during warmups.

"How've ya been, Bird Cage?" the Flags Captain asked me as we stood on the ice waiting for Eneman to drop the ceremonial puck.

"Having the time of my life!" I smiled.

When Eneman dropped the puck, I gently pulled it back to myself, picked it up and handed it back to him.

"I see you've finally learned how to take a ceremonial faceoff, eh?"

I rolled my eyes. "I'm telling my new team that you guys are picking on me," I laughed.

"It's all good, Bird Cage," he said with a smile before we skated back to our respective benches.

The Wings won the game, and I went back to the hotel to get some much-needed sleep.

On Sunday morning, I drove two and a half hours to the Allen County War Memorial Coliseum in Fort Wayne, Indiana. There was no practice that morning, so I took my time, arriving just after lunch. As soon as I pulled into the parking lot, my mouth fell open. Even from the outside, it was easy to tell that the Coliseum would be better suited for an NHL team, but once inside, I gasped when I stepped onto the Komets' bench and looked up, up, up. The arena must have held at least 14,000 people. Intimidating, to say the least.

An hour before the warmups, I dressed in my locker room and waited until I heard a knock at the door.

"Yes?" I said.

"Coach is ready for you to come in," one of my teammates said without opening the door.

I followed him into the nearly silent Komets' locker room, where the coach pointed sternly at an empty seat for me.

The coach turned and wildly drew on the chalkboard at the front of the locker room, spewing talk of systems and plays that were all well over my head. Then suddenly he threw the chalk down on the floor, looked directly at me and said loudly, "What's your name?"

"Molly," I practically whispered.

"Speak up!" he yelled.

"Molly," I said again, only slightly louder.

"And what are you here for?" he asked. I promptly explained why there was some chick, suited up and ready to play, in their locker room.

"I was diagnosed with colon cancer on my 23rd birthday and I'm here to skate with you guys tonight to raise awareness of colon cancer." I looked around the room and watched as the players seemed to relax a bit.

"In honor of Molly skating with us tonight, we're going to do a little cheer," the coach said. I looked around, confused. The player next to me just nodded his head and smiled.

"This half of the room," Coach said, waving his hand over the right side of the locker room, "when I say so, you're going to yell, 'Stick it!'" The guys all nodded in unison while I sat utterly perplexed. "This half of the room," he continued, waving his hand over the other side of the locker room, "you're going to yell, 'Pound it!'" More nodding in unison. "And you're going to say, 'Sexy!'" He pointed to a player in the corner.

"Got it," the lone player said. And before I knew it, the locker room had erupted with shouting as the coach waved his hand over the right side of the room.

"Stick it!" they yelled.

"Pound it," I joined in when he waved his hand over our side of the room.

"Sexy," the guy in the corner said.

Coach shook his head. "Not sexy enough. Do it again!"

I was mortified.

"Stick it!" the right side yelled.

"Pound it!" I yelled with my side of the room again.

"Sex-ay-y-y-y" the lone player growled.

"Way to go!" Coach said, and without another word, he walked out of the locker room, slamming the door behind him and leaving me in the middle of the laughter. I wasn't sure if I had just been sexually harassed, or if it was his way of keeping their spirits up. Either way, I liked him. He was funny, and I wasn't nervous.

On the ice, during the 20-minute pregame warmup, the team chanted as they passed the puck around. Whoever received it yelled, "Stick it!" The next to get it would yell, "Pound it!" Then, off in the distance I heard "Sex-ay-y-y-y!" It went on for the entire warmup and somehow I felt right at home.

When it was finally time to get on the ice for the game, I joined the Komets for a few laps while the music played.

"Hey Bird Cage!" I heard across the ice. "We miss you!" I smiled. It would be my last meeting with the Port Huron Flags, and I felt a twinge of sadness knowing that it would all be over soon.

"And now it's time for your starting lineup." The announcer's voice boomed through the immense arena. I followed the other Komets starters to the goal line and one-by-one, the announcer named them before each one skated to the blue line with applause. Finally, I stood alone.

"Now, please join me in welcoming the first female Komet in history to our starting lineup: Molly-y-y-y McMaster-r-r-r!" I looked up at the crowd. The massive arena wasn't full, but the crowd of nearly 7,000 seemed huge, and to my surprise every single one of them was on their feet. I took a deep breath and blinked away tears. I had completed a lot of firsts already that month, and a standing ovation was now on the list, but I didn't want to take home the honor of first to cry on the blue line. As the national anthem played, I willed away the tears.

The game puck dropped promptly at five p.m., and I had the longest shift of my UHL career, clocking in at a full minute and 13 seconds.

After the game, I joined my teammates in my first Post-Game Fan Skate, and there, a little girl wearing a Komets' jersey who couldn't have been more than 10 approached me.

"Can I have your autograph?" she asked sweetly.

"Sure," I said smiling. "Do you play hockey?" I signed the card and handed it back to her.

"Yeah," she said, "and I'm mad at you."

"Oh, yeah?" I looked up. "Why's that?"

"'Cause I wanted to be the first girl Komet."

Maybe Dad buying me hammers for Christmas all those years hadn't been such a bad thing after all. Maybe it had been his subtle way of telling me that it didn't matter that I was a girl. I could and *should* do anything I wanted. With one sentence, a pig-tailed, 10-year-old girl had just shown me that my skating with the UHL was reaching out in more ways than I had even considered.

On Monday, I flew to St. Louis, excited to practice with the Missouri River Otters for two days before the game on Wednesday night, but looking even more forward to visiting old friends and new.

After practice on Tuesday, I visited Tammy, one of our original 2005 Colondar models – the soccer player – and her beautiful new baby boy. It was simply awesome to see her living her dream of becoming a mom, something she didn't think she would be able to do after rectal cancer.

Then on Wednesday morning after practice, I bought a bottle of champagne and drove into St. Louis to sit with another survivor while he received his final chemotherapy treatment. Dr. Jeff, as we called him, was a radiologist who had already been chosen to pose for the 2007 Colondar, and he was being treated at the very hospital where he worked. I watched the chemo drug drip into his IV line and slide down through the tube and then underneath his shirt to his port. As we talked, I couldn't help but see myself there in a pink recliner identical to his. It was so hard to fathom that seven years had passed since I had sat in that chair. Seven years had passed since I had heard the words, "You have colon cancer."

That night, I suited up with the River Otters and then joined Tammy and her husband at the education table, along with several gastroenterology nurses. This was one of the many arenas where our growing number of Colondar models came out to share their stories and help educate about colorectal cancer. Our network was on the rise.

I flew to Chicago the following morning and drove on to Rockford, Illinois. When the IceHogs coach invited me to practice for the next two days, I jumped at the chance. March would be over soon, and I wanted to squeeze every last second out of it.

I woke up the next morning when it was still dark and drove to a local radio station to do an interview. Then I drove to the rink and went to the coach's office to introduce myself. I found him on the phone, but he waved me in anyway, so I tiptoed in and sat down, having no idea what was unfolding before me.

"I don't know. Let me ask her," he said to the person on the other end of the phone line. "Molly, do you want to play in tonight's game against the Vipers?"

"I thought I wasn't on with you guys until tomorrow," I said.

"That's alright. What do you say?"

"Heck, yeah!" I said.

"She said yes," he said into the receiver.

I practiced with the IceHogs that morning as planned, and learned that the local newspaper had run an article quoting the Viper's very large enforcer, the very same one who had visited my locker room before my game with the Frostbite a few weeks earlier. His message for the Rockford coach that morning was full of taunts and digs so, not to be outdone, the coach had his own interview with the same two disc jockeys that had interviewed me that very morning. That had been the call I walked in on. His plan was to match me up with the big guy every time he set foot on the ice, and he would donate $100 to The Colon Club for every shift I got. My job was simply to skate circles around him.

The game against the Vipers turned out to be all hype when the big guy never touched the ice after the warm-up. I never saw any ice either, but I didn't care. When I had arrived at the rink that night, instead of finding my jersey and equipment hanging in a private locker room, I was stunned when I walked into the *team* locker room and found my *very own* locker with my *very own* nameplate. My jersey hung with "McMaster" facing out and all my gear was put out just like everyone else's. I was one of them, if only for a few days. I didn't want to wake from my dream.

I practiced with the IceHogs again the following morning and joined them in their locker room again that night. I had learned early in the month about tacking money on the cork board for the player who scored the game-winner, and knowing that we would be facing off against *my* Frostbite, I came prepared. I waited until all the players were in their seats before walking over to the board with a crisp $100 bill in my hand. Then I held it up to the board and dramatically slammed a tack through it as my teammates hooted and whistled. I was an IceHog that night and I wanted them to know it.

The IceHogs won the game, and I was out a hundred bucks, but Rockford had been the best arena to date. The building had been full and electric. After the first period, I joined two 2006 Colondar models at the education table on the concourse, where the three of us shared our stories for hours with eager fans.

As the long autograph line began to fade, I felt a little sad. The month was ending soon, and I would be going back to my reality.

On Wednesday, March 22, with only two games left, I traded my helmet and "bird cage" for a Frostbite jersey and heavy camera makeup. I sat in a cold dark studio with a lone cameraman and on the screen in front of me, live and via satellite was Dana Jacobson of ESPN's *Cold Pizza*.

"Sundance College Hoops may be the fun part of March," Dana began on the screen in front of me, "but the month also has a serious theme. It is devoted to raising awareness about a disease that kills someone in the U.S. every nine minutes. I'm talking about colon cancer, and it's the disease Molly McMaster was diagnosed with when she was just 23."

Dana disappeared from the screen, and in her place was a video of me lifting weights and then suiting up in the Frostbite locker room.

"Now, seven years later, she is cancer-free and raising awareness by playing hockey on every team in the United Hockey League. She's got two more to go and she took some time off to join us this morning along with ESPN's Barry Melrose, who some of you may not know is also a team owner in the UHL."

The video on the screen disappeared and switched to a split screen where Barry and I were side by side.

"Molly, how'd you come up with this idea?" Dana asked me.

I told Dana about my conversation with Coach Potvin, and how the UHL commissioner had taken it a step further, asking me to play with all 14 teams to raise awareness of colorectal cancer.

"This is, by far, the best thing I've ever gotten the opportunity to do. I get to play professional hockey and raise awareness of colon cancer at the same time. It's just awesome!"

"You're obviously having an impact on raising awareness with the players," Dana said. "What's been the reaction though, out on the ice when you get added to their roster?"

"I've been pushed around a little bit," I laughed. "I can't really tell if the guys are flirting with me or what. I haven't been hit too hard yet though. They want to see me score."

"Barry," Dana shifted to him. "You're the owner of a team. You're Molly's *boss*." Barry laughed, and I rolled my eyes. "So, what's been the reaction around the league? What are you hearing from people out there?"

"Molly's got a passion for this," Barry began. "Molly wants to see an end to colon cancer. She wants to find a cure for every cancer. And I think the biggest thing is that every team has players that were touched by someone who has died of cancer. Molly's passionate about this. Hockey is a passionate sport. They realize why Molly's doing it, the courage it takes to go into the locker rooms of men, travel all over North America and do this night in and night out --- how hard it is. You don't travel first class in the United Hockey League." We all laughed. "The effort she's putting into it, the players respond to that."

I smiled.

"Did she ask you if you've had your colonoscopy yet?" Barry asked.

"No," Dana said.

"That's her big thing," he continued. "You've gotta have that as soon as you meet Molly," he said. I laughed, remembering how I had pestered him at the golf tournament the first time we met, and at every Frostbite game he'd attended since.

"Barry, have you had a colonoscopy?" Dana asked.

"No, but Molly bugs me about it every time I talk to her."

"Barry, you've gotta have one," she nagged. "Now, Molly, what are some of the symptoms that we should be looking for?"

"They say the most common symptom is no symptom at all, which is why you need to get screened when you turn 50, no matter *what* you think your body needs. Other symptoms are changes in your bowel habits, unexplained weight loss, vomiting, lack of energy, abdominal pain, all of those kinda gross things that you don't want to talk about, you don't want to think about. And if you have more than one of those for a couple of weeks, you need to go see a doctor and you need to get screened. This is a disease that can happen to anyone. It doesn't matter how old you are. It doesn't matter what skin color you have. It doesn't matter what your dog's name is. Everybody's at risk for colon cancer. It's the second leading cause of cancer death in the United States, and yet one of the only ones that we can actually test for and remove before it starts, just by getting a colonoscopy."

"Dana, you've gotta ask Molly about her hockey card," Barry interrupted. "She's got the greatest hockey card in the *world*." My cheeks instantly felt warm.

"Really? What is that, Molly?"

"Well," I started.

"C'mon, Molly," Barry teased. "Spill the beans."

"It's a bikini photo of me from a calendar that we turned into a hockey card," I said. "On the back it has the symptoms and risk factors of colorectal cancer. We were looking for something that the crowds would pick up and actually walk out of the arena with and um," I blushed again, "*that* does it."

"Oh, they're picking it up, alright," Barry teased again.

"Barry, we've got it right here," Dana said. I watched her hold my Colondar photo up to the camera. Barry laughed. "Molly, I'm pretty sure the guys are probably picking this one up," she said. "All the guys in the studio are staring right now."

"That's the idea. I'm taking one for the team on this one." I loved Barry's boisterous laugh.

"Thank you both for joining us. Molly, thank you for raising awareness and we're glad to hear again that you're cancer-free."

In front of me, the screen went dark and it hit me hard. Not only was the UHL Cross-Checks Colon Cancer reaching into UHL hockey arenas across the Midwest and Northeast, but now it was reaching sports fans across the entire country. Once again, we had gotten colons into a place they didn't belong.

"You're clear," the cameraman announced, bringing me back to the cold and dark room.

I looked up. "Thanks," I said.

I had butterflies in my stomach.

Two days later, I boarded my last outgoing flight for Richmond, Virginia, where I would face off against my own Frostbite again on Saturday night, a rematch of my first UHL appearance, but I would stand at the other end of the ice this time.

When we lined up at the faceoff dot to start the game, I immediately recognized the Adirondack power play line, but before I could blink, the ref had dropped the puck and we were already racing into our defensive end. Rapper, one of the larger Frostbite defensemen, went into the corner with one of the RiverDogs and I plowed in behind him. Despite being at least half a foot shorter, I cross-checked him hard in the back and attempted to hold him against the boards while my fellow RiverDog pulled the puck out and skated toward the Adirondack end. Rapper wheeled around, ready to pummel whoever held the stick that was in his back, but laughed when he realized it was me. I let out a grateful sigh and skated away.

My shift ended, and my plus/minus remained at zero. I left the rink with Hannah, who had come to the Virginia leg of the journey. We drove nearly until dawn to reach Roanoke, where I would play my last game in the United Hockey League that night.

When we arrived at the Roanoke Civic Center, the coach told me that they were running a short bench due to injuries. The Vipers were in last place in the league and had no chance of making the playoffs, so I begged him to let me play more than one shift. He never said yes, but he never said no either.

The arena was hardly packed when I was sent out as a center to take the opening face-off. I laughed when I made eye contact with the ref, knowing I was finally about to get my name on the score sheet. He winked at me and smiled back.

The unknowing Elmira Jackals centerman and I both bent over the face off dot on our respective sides, but I never broke eye contact with the ref as I pulled my right hand from my glove and held my thumb and index fingers about two inches apart.

"Your thing is this big," I whispered to the referee.

"You have to speak up for the crowd," he said, unable to contain his laughter.

The Elmira Jackals centerman began to convulse with laughter, unaware that the referee and I had planned this scene out when I'd arrived at the arena that afternoon.

"You're thing is this big," I repeated a little bit more confidently.

The ref, doing everything in his power to hold a straight face, stood up, dropped the puck on the faceoff dot, blew his whistle, and put both hands on his waist to signal a misconduct penalty.

"Number six! Two minutes for unsportsmanlike conduct!" he yelled with a smirk and then nodded his head toward the box. "Now you go feel shame."

I laughed all the way across the ice. After getting on the ice with 14 teams that month, I would finally and officially get my name on the score sheet.

When my penalty was over, I skated across the ice to the Vipers bench and got a few high-fives before sitting down and realizing that I had just given up my one shift to sit in the box. Seeing that the game was getting rough, I convinced myself that it was better that way, but within a few minutes, one of the Vipers got a two-minute penalty. Instead of serving it, he simply left the ice.

"Someone needs to serve it, Coach," the referee said as he skated by the bench.

"I'll do it!" I piped up, more excited than anyone should ever be to spend time in the penalty box.

"Go for it," the coach said, and I hopped over the boards. I watched the game from the box again and when my two minutes were up and I was sprung, I skated as hard as I could across the ice to the Roanoke bench for one of the Vipers to take my place. Instead, I found the coach waving me away.

"Stay out there," he yelled at me, and I gladly did, putting a solid effort into my final minute on the ice in the UHL.

Later that night, when I joined the team as they celebrated their first win in a long time, I was pulled aside by one of the players.

"I lost my sister in a car accident a few years ago," he said.

"I'm so sorry," I responded, not sure what to say.

"I felt like my world ended," he continued, "but you have shown me that you can take something so bad and turn it into something so good." He smiled. "Thank you for doing what you do."

For what felt like the millionth time, I was stunned.

The month of March 2006 had been a dream come true. I had joined an elite group of only five or six women in the world who were able to say they had played men's professional hockey. Of those women, I was the only one who hadn't played for a national team, let alone a collegiate team. The only other woman who had played in the UHL was Erin Whitten, a goalie who had played on the boys' hockey team at -- ironically -- my high school.

The UHL Cross-Checks Colon Cancer was an incredible success, and the most amazing and rewarding part of the experience was bringing colorectal cancer education into an arena where the stereotype was the pizza-eating, beer-guzzling sports fan who knew nothing about colon cancer. These people learned about the disease because Eneman and I were at their arena for one night in the month of March, and we were able to show the fans that colon cancer can happen to anyone.

26

SURPRISE!

After my month-long UHL tour, I arrived home on an absolute high, but utterly exhausted. Jetting off to Maui, Hawaii with Sergei for a week was a welcome break. We ate. We slept. We played golf and went snorkeling. We lay on the beach and took in the scenery.

Just before the UHL playoffs were set to begin, we landed back in New York to learn that the fifth seeded Adirondack Frostbite had clinched a spot.

At the end of each of the UHL games in March, I had the teams autograph my jerseys, which we then auctioned on eBay, raising nearly $5,000 for The Colon Club. All the teams had been fun, but the Muskegon Fury was by far my favorite. I didn't tell anyone, but I had bid on and won my Muskegon jersey, and had it hanging on the back of my office chair at home. Imagine my excitement when I learned that *my* Fury would be coming to town to face the Frostbite in round one of the playoffs.

The series began with Adirondack traveling to Muskegon only to lose games one and two on the road. Then it was time for games three and four at home. I was thrilled that I would see *my* Fury. Apparently, they were looking forward to seeing me, too.

"Hello?" I said, looking at the clock. It was 10:30 on a Wednesday night, two days before game three and I was struggling to keep my eyes open.

"*Who* is Jason Lawmaster?" my mother asked sharply, and I started to laugh. "He just called here looking for you, and I heard loud hooting in the background," she said. "Apparently they went through the phone book and called all the McMasters asking for you until they found us."

The next morning, I crawled out of bed and made my way to the rink in time for their practice, plopping myself down in a chair in the middle of their locker room.

"Missed you guys," I said with a huge smile. Once again, they welcomed me in, and I felt right at home.

The Fury came up short in game three, proving I was no longer their lucky charm, but they invited me to join them out after the game anyway. I didn't stay late. During the game, I had been so tired that I went into the office more than once to rest. I didn't know what was wrong.

After game four and the Fury's second loss, I said goodbye as they loaded their bus for the long, overnight drive back to Michigan. Meanwhile, I was looking forward to a few days off. All I wanted to do was to crawl into bed, pull the covers over my head and sleep for days. On a whim, I stopped at the drugstore for a pregnancy test. An hour later, Sergei and I were staring at a faint blue line.

When I sat in the examining room on the crinkling paper that I had become so familiar with, I smiled. For the first time in a long time, this doctor's appointment had nothing to do with cancer. There was a knock on the door, and my sister-in-law, Aimee, walked in.

"What's going on today? Says here that you need a physical?"

"Not exactly," I said. "Aimee, right now, you're my nurse practitioner and not my sister-in-law, OK? That means everything in this room stays in this room, right?"

"Yes," she said. Aimee looked concerned and took a seat on the rolling doctor stool.

"Good," I smiled. "I think I might be pregnant."

"You suck!" she said, and I laughed, knowing that she legally couldn't say anything to the family or anyone else.

Aimee took some blood from my arm, tested it, and then gave me the news.

"You're about five or six weeks along," she said.

We chatted for few minutes about how I was feeling and then about my brother, my niece who was nearly three, and both of my nephews.

"How has Timmy been doing?" I asked of the nephew who had been diagnosed with Ewing's Sarcoma during the Colossal Colon Tour.

"He's already planning his third annual Tim's Bears Who Care Day," Aimee told me. I couldn't believe that a seventh-grader had the compassion and drive to put together a project like he had. "He and some of his classmates have already raised enough money to build 100 bears this year!" After they raised the money, they would go to the Build-A-Bear Workshop, create the bears, and then donate them to the Albany Medical Center's Pediatric Hematology/Oncology unit where they were given to kids who were diagnosed with cancer so they didn't have to "go through it alone."

"He is lucky to have another survivor like you to look up to," Aimee said.

She gave me a big hug and congratulated me as I left the doctor's office.

When I got into my car, I put the key into the ignition but just sat there, staring into space. For seven years, I had no idea if I would be able to get pregnant after having cancer and chemotherapy. Now it was happening.

A few days later, the Frostbite got knocked out of the playoffs by the Fury after losing games five and six in Muskegon, ending their season, but it didn't much matter. I would be taking a break from hockey for a little while.

"Do you want a boy or a girl?" I asked Sergei over dinner one night.

"I want a healthy baby," he said.

"I know that, but if you had a choice, would you choose a boy or a girl?"

"I can't answer that," he said. "Can you?"

"Point taken." I smirked at him. "I get to be the hockey coach though," I added.

"No way! Why?"

"Because I have been teaching people how to ice skate and coaching for almost 10 years."

"So," he said. I've been playing for twice as long."

"*So*," I said sarcastically.

We both dug in our heels.

"OK," I said, "how about this? If we have a boy, you can coach. If we have a girl, I get to coach." I wasn't thrilled with this idea, but I was so certain there was a baby girl in my belly that I was willing to risk it.

"Deal," he finally said. The line had been drawn.

As the first trimester rolled along and my belly began to pudge, I grew anxious about my pregnancy, as most mothers-to-be do. I worried about the baby being healthy and about being a good mother, but I was also scared of how the birthing process would go, especially if any scar tissue or adhesions had developed after my two abdominal surgeries. I was also afraid of complications if I had to have a C-section. At my next appointment, my midwife was unconcerned. "Women with Crohn's disease and women who have undergone similar surgeries have babies all the time without any trouble," she said. I wasn't convinced. She didn't have any solid statistics about women who had given birth after colon cancer, so I began looking into it myself.

A few months before learning I was pregnant, I had posed a question about adhesions and pregnancy on The Colon Club's message board, more for the other members than for myself. At that point, I had only heard of two women who had given birth after colon cancer. Both were 2005 Colondar models, and both responded to my post. Tammy's very positive experience with in-vitro fertilization resulted in a healthy baby boy, while Sara's doctor told her that adhesions caused her child to be born premature, at just over 24 weeks. At birth, her baby girl weighed just one pound and seven ounces.

No one else had responded to my post.

My pregnancy crept along, and I made it through the 2007 Colondar photo shoot purely on adrenaline. Once I was safely past my first trimester, my exhaustion finally passed. Then, at 18 weeks, right around the same time Troy was putting the finishing touches on the Colondar and getting ready to send it off to the printer, I was scheduled for an ultrasound. Sergei and I would find out the sex of our new baby and finally end the battle over who would coach the family hockey team.

At the obstetrician's office, I lay on a table in a dark room, with Sergei at my side, watching the screen in front of me. The ultrasound technician found the heartbeat and took the fetus' measurements. She rolled the cold and gooey wand all over my belly for an eternity before getting to the most important part.

"Looks like you'll be having a boy!" she said.

"*Dammit!*" I practically shouted. But I quickly realized the absurdity of my reaction. "I didn't mean it like that!" I said shaking my head and explaining our bet to the technician.

I still wasn't able to find out much about having babies after colon cancer and that had been weighing on my mind. I set up my next appointment with Dr. Roberts, or Mo as I had gotten to know her as a teammate on the ice, determined to get answers to my questions.

Mo asked me all the usual health questions until finally I heard the one I was waiting for.

"Do you have any concerns?"

"I do," I said. You know about my history and that I was diagnosed with colon cancer when I was 23. Since Dr. Martelo found out that I was pregnant, I've been seeing him monthly to keep an eye on my incision," I told her.

"That's a good idea," Mo said.

"I've asked him a little bit about what to expect, given my abdominal surgeries and chemo, but he hasn't really been able to give me a solid answer because he hasn't been able to find any other cases like mine --- women having babies after colon resections due to cancer. I also know that my second surgery was performed partly because of some adhesions that had formed. I'm scared about adhesions."

"Moll," Mo began, "I think you have every right to be nervous. I don't think anything is going to go wrong, based on the shape you are in, but why don't we put a sort of team together. I would be more than happy to get in touch with Dr. Martelo myself. I also recommend that you choose a surgeon to be on-call when you go into labor. That way, if there are any complications and you do need a C-Section, he will be there to assist, if needed."

"OK. That sounds good," I said.

"We'll keep a close eye on you," she promised.

I left the office feeling much better about the proactive role I was taking in my pregnancy. I made an appointment with a surgeon and called Dr. Alexander Parikh, a friend and surgical oncologist at Vanderbilt-Ingram Cancer Center, to get another opinion.

"You're probably going to be fine," Dr. Parikh said. "I've assisted on C-sections after colon resections before, and the only time I've seen any complications was in patients where mesh was used in their colectomy to reduce the formation of adhesions. Do you know if your surgeon used mesh?" he asked.

"I don't know, but I have my surgical records. I'll look through them and find out."

Dr. Parikh answered every neurotic question I could think of with the patience of a preschool teacher. We hung up and I poured through my surgical reports, relieved to find that, Dr. Thompson had not used mesh.

The baby continued to grow inside of me, and by the time I was into my third trimester, my team of doctors was set up, each caring for me in a different way. I was finally feeling more in control.

Meanwhile, my work with The Colon Club went on. The Colossal Colon still toured smaller, private venues around the country, even trekking all the way to Alaska by barge and, after a brief holdup at the border, making an international appearance in Montreal, Canada. Hannah, Troy and I madly worked to finish the 2007 Colondar and promote it nationwide, and I continued to answer emails daily from hockey fans, patients, and people with symptoms who were too scared to tell their doctor.

September 14, 2006

Molly,

Thank you very much for the 2007 Colondar. It is certainly a magnificent piece of work.

Your efforts at organizing something like this and your determination to raise colon cancer awareness has saved many lives already. You probably just don't hear about those cases.

I read somewhere a long time ago that the best thing you could do with your life is to spend it doing something that will outlast it. You're a perfect example of that. It's just that I'm sure you need to hear that once in a while.

From now on, whenever someone says one person can make a difference, I'll be thinking of you.

> *All the best,*
> *Peter Pepe*

My belly continued to grow into the final weeks and exhaustion took hold again, but I still jumped at the chance to get back on the ice and help coach a kids' hockey clinic for a few days. Since I obviously wasn't going to be playing until after the baby was born, coaching would have to do. It really did feel wonderful to be back on the ice, so when a 10-year-old boy bragged that he was faster than me, I raced around with him a few times to prove him wrong.

Two weeks after coaching the hockey clinic, and four days before my due date, Sergei and I went into the hospital. At 1:07 a.m. on Christmas Eve 2006, Kyril James Morgoslepov was born without any complications and without the need for a surgeon. I held him in my arms, and for the first time, I truly understood the meaning of love at first sight. Looking into his beautiful blue eyes, I couldn't imagine that only a few years earlier I had been in so much pain that I had considered ending it all.

Life with a baby wasn't anything like what I had expected. Sergei and I did not leave the house for the first four days, and if Mom hadn't stayed with us, we probably wouldn't have had anything to eat. Then there were the emotions. My heart tightened whenever I thought about anyone caring for Kyril but me. Suddenly, daycare seemed out of the question. We had him for less than a week, but Kyril was already our little dictator.

"I never knew you could love something so much," I said to Sergei, "not that I don't love *you*."

"I know," he said. "I love you too, but it is different. It's unconditional."

I knew exactly what he meant. It *was* unconditional.

Ten days after arriving home from the hospital, I got a call from my assistant coach with the Adirondack Empire State Women's Ice Hockey team. It was the first time I had thought about anything *but* taking care of Kyril since he'd come into my world.

"Molly! Tryouts are this weekend! Are you coming?" he asked.

"Um," I stalled. "Probably not. I just had a baby!"

"You can skate," he said. "Come to the tryout. All you need to do is get on the ice. And that is the first reason I was calling. The second is to say thank you."

"For what?" I asked.

"I've had your hockey card in my car ever since you gave it to me."

"The "*dirty*" hockey card?" I teased.

"Yes," he continued in a voice that sounded serious. "I had a physical recently and since I was having some bleeding, I told my doctor that I thought I needed a colonoscopy. He said I was too young, but I told him about you, so he sent me for one. I had more than 20 polyps removed. Molly, you saved my life."

I was speechless and reminded once again that until the last person in the world heard the words, "You have colon cancer," I would always have a promise to keep. Kyril would just have to get used to listening to his mommy talk about colons.

EPILOGUE

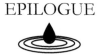

In 1999, on the morning that Dr. Thompson told me I had colon cancer, my life suddenly looked bleak. But my biggest fear wasn't the cancer, the chemo or even my own demise. My biggest fear was that all the confidence and strength I had finally found in Colorado would be shattered, and I would forever be known as "poor little Molly with cancer." Standing on the edge of that cliff was my test. Would I *have* cancer? Or would I *fight* it? I had to make a choice.

I could never begin to fathom the possibilities that could follow after simply choosing confidence and strength, beginning with Rolling to Recovery in 2000. Strangers across the country followed and supported the crusade, and back home the entire North Country held me up.

The online guestbook that Sergei created so long ago for Rolling to Recovery became a support group for me as I skated across the country. I had no idea that others were also using it to find support through one another, beginning one of the first online support groups for colorectal cancer. Since then, the guest book has morphed into Colon Talk, The Colon Club's online forum where new patients, survivors and caregivers can connect and ask questions as they enter their own journey.

In 2010, exactly 10 years after I started my skate from Glens Falls to the West in the spitting rain, a young man named Andrew Hudon who had read about Rolling to Recovery decided that he too wanted to make a difference. Andrew began his own journey --- by bicycle --- riding from Colorado to Glens Falls to raise money and awareness of cancer. The Resilience Ride.

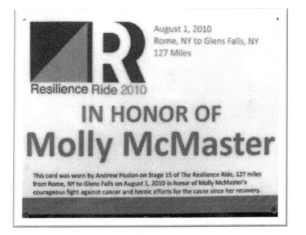

Card Worn by Andrew Hudon During the Resilience Ride

To the original cross-
Country badass! Thank
you for your friendship
and for inspiring me
and so many others!
- Drew

Back of Card Worn by Andrew Hudon During the Resilience Ride

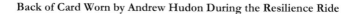

At the last mile of Andrew's journey, I handed him a set of dog tags with the inscription "one drop of rain ripples an entire pond," before skating the final mile with him. Two years later, he wore them when he rode coast to coast to raise more money and more awareness.

When Andrew finished that ride, his doctor warned that his knee was near ruin and he should never ride again, but his crusade continued. He took up swimming, and in 2014, in 20 hours, over two days, he swam 32 miles, from one end of Lake George to the other, to raise money for The Colon Club and the Colon Cancer Alliance. Andrew called his event "The Ripple Effect."

Today, those ripples have become raging swells as more and more survivors and their supporters work together to raise awareness. The Colon Club is an army of hundreds of survivors all over the country, many of whom have posed for the Colondar and *On the Rise* magazine. The photo shoot is now run nearly entirely by volunteers, many of whom once stood bravely under the bright lights, sharing their scars and baring their souls. Today they help create the experience for the next group of survivor advocates.

After the magic dust has been sprinkled, survivors are challenged to raise awareness of colorectal cancer in their own hometowns, furthering the mission of The Colon Club. *On the Rise* models are also introduced to other colorectal cancer organizations so they can become involved in the one that speaks to them. Each survivor decides how to create their own ripples.

In the past few years, at the *On the Rise* photo shoots, I've had the honor of watching in awe as the magic happens all over again, and the ripples continue to grow.

If it wasn't for The Colon Club, I would have never found the strength and confidence to grow into the empowered advocate that I am today. It may have taken me 15 years to get here, but I'm going to be loud and proud for the rest of my days.

My second shout out is to the Colorectal Cancer Alliance. I want to grow with your organization as well. Thank you for giving me another avenue to learn, grow and advocate. Be your own advocate, get more than one opinion, demand to be screened if you are experiencing any symptoms. Colorectal cancer is preventable, treatable and beatable.

Denelle Wirth Suranski
2019 On the Rise Model (via Facebook)

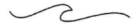

Today, the Colossal Colon is permanently at home in the Health Museum in Houston, still doing her job by educating hundreds of visitors every day. Inspired by CoCo, educational blow-up colons are now appearing all over the world.

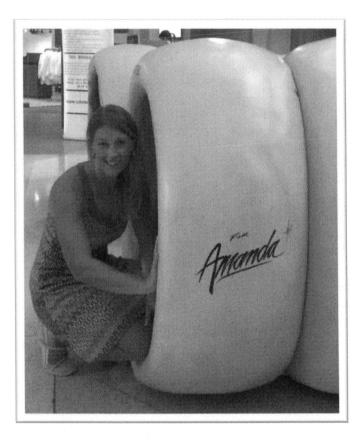

CoCo at the Health Museum

On February 22, 2008, nearly five years after Dave Barry wrote his column about the Colossal Colon during its national tour in 2003, I opened another newspaper to find that he had written a second column for the Miami Herald about colon cancer.

A Journey into My Colon — and Yours

BY DAVE BARRY

OK. You turned 50. You know you're supposed to get a colonoscopy. But you haven't. Here are your reasons:

1. You've been busy.

2. You don't have a history of cancer in your family.

3. You haven't noticed any problems.

4. You don't want a doctor to stick a tube 17,000 feet up your butt.

Let's examine these reasons one at a time. No, wait, let's not. Because you and I both know that the only real reason is No. 4. This is natural. The idea of having another human, even a medical human, becoming deeply involved in what is technically known as your "behindular zone" gives you the creeping willies.

I know this because I am like you, except worse. I yield to nobody in the field of being a pathetic weenie medical coward. I become faint and nauseous during even very minor medical procedures, such as making an appointment by phone. It's much worse when I come into physical contact with the medical profession. More than one doctor's office has a dent in the floor caused by my forehead striking it seconds after I got a shot.

In 1997, when I turned 50, everybody told me I should get a colonoscopy. I agreed that I definitely should, but not right away. By following this policy, I reached age 55 without having had a colonoscopy. Then I did something so pathetic and embarrassing that I am frankly ashamed to tell you about it.

What happened was, a giant 40-foot replica of a human colon came to Miami Beach. Really. It's an educational exhibit called the Colossal Colon, and it was on a nationwide tour to promote awareness of colorectal cancer. The idea is, you crawl through the Colossal Colon, and you encounter various educational items in there, such as polyps, cancer and hemorrhoids the size of regulation volleyballs, and you go, "Whoa, I better find out if I contain any of these things," and you get a colonoscopy.

If you are as a professional humor writer, and there is a giant colon within a 200-mile radius, you are legally obligated to go see it. So I went to Miami Beach and crawled through the Colossal Colon. I wrote a column about it, making tasteless colon jokes. But I also urged everyone to get a colonoscopy. I even, when I emerged from the Colossal Colon, signed a pledge stating that I would get one.

But I didn't get one. I was a fraud, a hypocrite, a liar. I was practically a member of Congress.

Five more years passed. I turned 60, and I still hadn't gotten a colonoscopy. Then, a couple of weeks ago, I got an e-mail from my brother Sam, who is 10 years younger than I am, but more mature. The email was addressed to me and my middle brother, Phil. It said:

``Dear Brothers,

``I went in for a routine colonoscopy and got the dreaded diagnosis: cancer. We're told it's early and that there is a good prognosis that they can get it all out, so, fingers crossed, knock on wood, and all that. And of course they told me to tell my siblings to get screened. I imagine you both have."

Um. Well.

First I called Sam. He was hopeful, but scared. We talked for a while, and when we hung up, I called my friend Andy Sable, a gastroenterologist, to make an appointment for a colonoscopy. A few days later, in his office, Andy showed me a color diagram of the colon, a lengthy organ that appears to go all over the place, at one point passing briefly through Minneapolis. Then Andy explained the colonoscopy procedure to me in a thorough, reassuring and patient manner. I nodded thoughtfully, but I didn't really hear anything he said, because my brain was shrieking, quote, ``HE'S GOING TO STICK A TUBE 17,000 FEET UP YOUR BUTT!"

I left Andy's office with some written instructions, and a prescription for a product called "MoviPrep," which comes in a box large enough to hold a microwave oven. I will discuss MoviPrep in detail later; for now suffice it to say that we must never allow it to fall into the hands of America's enemies.

I spent the next several days productively sitting around being nervous. Then, on the day before my colonoscopy, I began my preparation. In accordance with my instructions, I didn't eat any solid food that day; all I had was chicken broth, which is basically water, only with less flavor. Then, in the evening, I took the MoviPrep. You mix two packets of powder together in a one-liter plastic jug, then you fill it with lukewarm water. (For those unfamiliar with the metric system, a liter is about 32 gallons.) Then you have to drink the whole jug. This takes about an hour, because MoviPrep tastes -- and here I am being kind -- like a mixture of goat spit and urinal cleanser, with just a hint of lemon.

The instructions for MoviPrep, clearly written by somebody with a great sense of humor, state that after you drink it, "a loose watery bowel movement may result." This is kind of like saying that after you jump off your roof, you may experience contact with the ground.

MoviPrep is a nuclear laxative. I don't want to be too graphic, here, but: Have you ever seen a space shuttle launch? This is pretty much the MoviPrep experience, with you as the shuttle. There are times when you wish the commode had a seat belt. You spend several hours pretty much confined to the bathroom, spurting violently. You eliminate everything. And then, when you figure you must be totally empty, you have to drink another liter of MoviPrep, at which point, as far as I can tell, your bowels travel into the future and start eliminating food that you have not even eaten yet.

After an action-packed evening, I finally got to sleep. The next morning my wife drove me to the clinic. I was very nervous. Not only was I worried about the procedure, but I had been experiencing occasional return bouts of MoviPrep spurtage. I was thinking, "What if I spurt on Andy?" How do you apologize to a friend for something like that? Flowers would not be enough.

At the clinic I had to sign many forms acknowledging that I understood and totally agreed with whatever the hell the forms said. Then they led me to a room full of other colonoscopy people, where I went inside a little curtained space and took off my clothes and put on one of those hospital garments designed by sadist perverts, the kind that, when you put it on, makes you feel even more naked than when you are actually naked.

Then a nurse named Eddie put a little needle in a vein in my left hand. Ordinarily I would have fainted, but Eddie was very good, and I was already lying down. Eddie also told me that some people put vodka in their MoviPrep. At first I was ticked off that I hadn't thought of this, but then I pondered what would happen if you got yourself too tipsy to make it to the bathroom, so you were staggering around in full Fire Hose Mode. You would have no choice but to burn your house.

When everything was ready, Eddie wheeled me into the procedure room, where Andy was waiting with a nurse and an anesthesiologist. I did not see the 17,000-foot tube, but I knew Andy had it hidden around there somewhere. I was seriously nervous at this point. Andy had me roll over on my left side, and the anesthesiologist began hooking something up to the needle in my hand. There was music playing in the room, and I realized that the song was Dancing Queen by Abba. I remarked to Andy that, of all the songs that could be playing during this particular procedure, Dancing Queen has to be the least appropriate.

"You want me to turn it up?" said Andy, from somewhere behind me.

"Ha ha," I said.

And then it was time, the moment I had been dreading for more than a decade. If you are squeamish, prepare yourself, because I am going to tell you, in explicit detail, exactly what it was like.

I have no idea. Really. I slept through it. One moment, Abba was shrieking ``Dancing Queen! Feel the beat from the tambourine . . ."

. . . and the next moment, I was back in the other room, waking up in a very mellow mood. Andy was looking down at me and asking me how I felt. I felt excellent. I felt even more excellent when Andy told me that it was all over, and that my colon had passed with flying colors. I have never been prouder of an internal organ.

But my point is this: In addition to being a pathetic medical weenie, I was a complete moron. For more than a decade I avoided getting a procedure that was, essentially, nothing. There was no pain and, except for the MoviPrep, no discomfort. I was risking my life for nothing.

If my brother Sam had been as stupid as I was -- if, when he turned 50, he had ignored all the medical advice and avoided getting screened -- he still would have had cancer. He just wouldn't have known. And by the time he did know -- by the time he felt symptoms -- his situation would have been much, much more serious. But because he was a grown-up, the doctors caught the cancer early, and they operated and took it out. Sam is now recovering and eating what he describes as "really, really boring food." His prognosis is good, and everybody is optimistic, fingers crossed, knock on wood, and all that.

Which brings us to you, Mr. or Mrs. or Miss or Ms. Over-50-And-Hasn't-Had-a-Colonoscopy. Here's the deal: You either have colorectal cancer, or you don't. If you do, a colonoscopy will enable doctors to find it and do something about it. And if you don't have cancer, believe me, it's very reassuring to know you don't. There is no sane reason for you not to have it done.

I am so eager for you to do this that I am going to induce you with an Exclusive Limited Time Offer. If you, after reading this, get a colonoscopy, let me know by sending a self-addressed stamped envelope to Dave Barry Colonoscopy Inducement, The Miami Herald, 3511 NW 91st Ave., Miami, FL, 33172. I will send you back a certificate, signed by me and suitable for framing if you don't mind framing a cheesy certificate, stating that you are a grown-up who got a colonoscopy. Accompanying this certificate will be a square of limited-edition custom-printed toilet paper with an image of Miss Paris Hilton on it. You may frame this also, or use it in whatever other way you deem fit.

But even if you don't want this inducement, please get a colonoscopy. If I can do it, you can do it. Don't put it off. Just do it.
Be sure to stress that you want the non-Abba version.

©2008 Dave Barry

Once again, Dave had created ripples of his own.

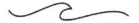

After drawing courage and strength from the necklace Sarah gave me so many years ago, I don't feel I *need* to wear it anymore, having come a long way from that insecure college kid with the screeching cat in her stomach at CSU. But I did eventually have the symbol tattooed on the inside of my left wrist so it would be with me forever. Call it superstition.

Sergei and I are happily married and the proud parents of two healthy and very active boys. Kyril's younger brother Maksim Vladimir was born on January 21, 2009 without complications. Sergei and I have also finally come to a coaching agreement. He has been kind enough to share duties with me by switching who coaches which boy each year. I am still playing hockey of course, but I now find it more fun to watch my children's passion for the sport.

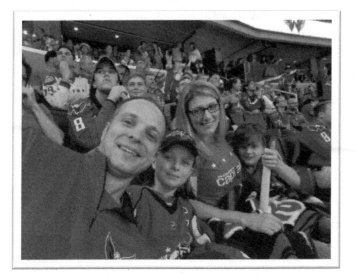

Sergei, Kyril, Me and Maks

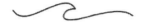

Jaws don't drop the way they used to when I tell someone that I was diagnosed with colon cancer at the age of 23, and the time finally came for me to step back from the day-today operation of The Colon Club. I knew that day would come and was terrified that it would cease to exist without me, having been the face for so long. Part of me also felt like I might be letting Amanda down, but what I have realized instead is that The Colon Club is rolling like a freight train now, and nothing can stop it.

The truth is, none of us will ever realize the full impact of our actions. We may never get to see the ripples that we create ourselves, but they are there. And every single one of us is capable of making them. That's another thing that makes me feel so lucky. I *have* seen many of those ripples.

Today, this movement – this legacy – is bigger than any of us, and as I look back on my life, I am humbled beyond words to realize that all it took to start the storm was a single drop of rain.

Symptoms of Colorectal Cancer

- The most common symptom is no symptom at all
- Change in bowel habits - diarrhea and/or constipation, narrow stools
- Unexplained weight loss, vomiting
- Anemia, lack of energy
- Blood, often not visible, in stool or from rectum
- Abdominal pain, and/or discomfort - gas, bloating, cramps, feeling that the bowel does not empty

If you have more than one of these symptoms for a few weeks, or if you have a family history of cancer, polyps, or other diseases of the colon, see a doctor and be persistent until you get an explanation.

The Colon Club seeks to educate as many people as possible, as early as possible, about the risk factors and symptoms of colorectal cancer, and encourages people to get screened when it's appropriate for them. To learn more about colorectal cancer, connect through COLON TALK, apply for the Kimberly Fund, and purchase Colon Swag, go to The Colon Club. **www.colonclub.com**

To Connect with The Colon Club on Facebook got to
www.facebook.com/colonclub/

To visit the **Colossal Colon**, go to:
The Health Museum
1515 Hermann Drive
Houston, TX 77004
Phone: 713-521-1515
www.thehealthmuseum.org

MORE RESOURCES:

Alive and Kickn seeks to improve the lives of individuals and families affected by Lynch syndrome and associated cancers through research, education and screening. **www.aliveandkickn.org**

The Blue Hat Foundation is a colorectal cancer organization whose mission is to educate, raise awareness, and provide resources to free screenings for minority and medically underserved communities. We work hard to take care of the neediest members of our community and provide them with unconditional support. **www.thebluehatfoundation.org**

Cancer*Care* provides free, professional support services for people affected by colorectal cancer, as well as colorectal cancer treatment information and additional resources. **www.cancercare.org**

Colon Cancer Coalition was started in 2004 when Kristin Lindquist started planning for the very first Get Your Rear in Gear® run after losing her best friend and sister, Susie Lindquist Mjelde, to colon cancer. What started as one women's vision has since grown into a national coalition of people determined to end colorectal cancer deaths by increasing screening and educating others about the signs and symptoms of this treatable disease. We want all people to understand their risk factors and get the right screening at the right time. **www.coloncancercoalition.org**

The Colon Cancer Foundation is dedicated to a world without colorectal cancer through awareness, prevention, screening, and research.
www.coloncancerfoundation.org

Colorectal Cancer Alliance seeks to empower a nation of allies working together to provide support for patients and families, caregivers, and survivors; to raise awareness of preventive measures; and inspire efforts to fund critical research. **www.ccalliance.org**

Colorectal Cancer Canada is dedicated to increasing awareness of colorectal cancer, supporting patients, and advocating on their behalf.
www.colorectalcancercanada.com

Fight Colorectal Cancer empowers and activates patients, fighters and champions to push for better policies and to support research, education and awareness for all those touched by this disease.
www.fightcolorectalcancer.org

Prevent Cancer Foundation® seeks to save lives across all populations through cancer prevention and early detection. **www.preventcancer.org**

United Ostomy Associations of America Inc. (UOAA) supports, empowers, and advocates for people who have had or who will have ostomy or continent diversion surgery. **www.ostomy.org**

ABOUT THE AUTHOR

Molly McMaster Morgoslepov was diagnosed with colon cancer at 23 and began raising awareness of the disease in "out-of-the-box ways." She has in-line skated from New York to Colorado, run the New York City Marathon and conceived of the Colossal Colon, a 40-foot-long, 4-foot-tall, crawl-through replica of a human colon. Molly also co-founded The Colon Club, a nonprofit organization dedicated to raising awareness of colorectal cancer, especially in young people.

Molly is an ACSM Certified Personal Trainer and USA Hockey Level 4 Coach. She is a partner in the Saratoga Ninja Lab and lives in upstate New York with her husband, Sergei, and their two sons, Kyril and Maks. She has been cancer-free for over 20 years.

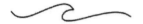

*This book is written about one survivor's experience and should in no way be taken as medical advice. Treatment options, surgical procedures, etc. have changed in the years since Molly was diagnosed with colon cancer. If you have symptoms, please see a doctor and get screened. If you have been diagnosed with colorectal cancer, please see the list of resources at the back of this book.

**Some character names have been changed.

Made in the
USA
Middletown, DE